IC Journey to Wellness

Healing Bladder Pain Syndrome and Interstitial Cystitis

Jill M. Peters-Gee, M.D.

www.icjourneytowellness.com

The material in this book is neither intended nor implied to be given as medical advice. I do not intend this publication to serve as a substitute for medical care or consultation with your physician or medical practitioner. This book should bring the reader up to date on current research and propose a new way of thinking about Interstitial Cystitis and Bladder Pain Syndrome. I have gathered the information contained from multiple sources intending to share this wide range of information. I have attempted to give proper credit to all sources. If you have additional questions, please consult your physician or medical practitioner.

I discuss various trademarked products and names in this book. I used these products editorially with no intention of infringement of the trademark. Copyright permission was granted for the use of the questionnaires used as resources in the toolbox at the end of the book.

Publishing Services provided by Paper Raven Books LLC
Printed in the United States of America
First Printing, 2024
Cover design by Chris Arrow, 99Designs

Paperback ISBN 979-8-9893651-0-4
Hardback ISBN 979-8-9893651-1-1

About the Cover

Embark on a transformative journey with me through the pages of this book, a journey that is necessary if you are living with Interstitial Cystitis or Bladder Pain Syndrome. This path is more than just a medical exploration; it is a journey of self-discovery. Together we will delve into your past experiences and your present symptoms, uncovering valuable clues that will lead you to defining and understanding your specific subtype or phenotype(s) of Interstitial Cystitis or Bladder Pain Syndrome.

Imagine the cover of this book—a winding path in Galicia, along the renowned Camino de Santiago in northern Spain. For over a millennium, this pilgrimage route has drawn millions of pilgrims from all walks of life. I count myself fortunate to have walked this path twice, in 2019 and again in 2023. The Camino is not just a physical journey; it's a profound exploration of the self. For some, it's a spiritual journey, while for others, it's a quest for answers, a means to heal from grief and loss, a celebration of life, a chance to explore new possibilities, or simply an opportunity to pause and reflect—a journey towards wellness.

The image of the well-trodden path on the cover represents a path of hope. It's a path where life is simplified, where you carry only the essentials in a modest backpack. Here, you learn to attune to your body's whispers and savor the beauty that surrounds you. This path has an extraordinary ability to heal, even when you might not have realized your soul needed healing. The light ahead symbolizes the hope that this book aspires to offer all those who read it. As we say on the Camino, "Buen Camino!"—wishing you a fulfilling and hopeful journey ahead.

Table of Contents

Part I

How Do You Know If You Have Interstitial Cystitis or Bladder Pain Syndrome?

As a urologist with over thirty years of experience treating patients, I have seen firsthand how Interstitial Cystitis (IC) and Bladder Pain Syndrome (BPS) can affect the lives of thousands of people. I have witnessed the frustration and difficulty that patients face in getting an accurate diagnosis and effective treatment. Clinicians can get equally frustrated, as they want to help, and sometimes it feels like no matter what they do, symptom relief is elusive. Interstitial cystitis and Bladder Pain Syndrome are complex conditions that can manifest with a variety of symptoms that are not always caused by bladder problems alone. This makes it challenging for clinicians to develop individualized treatment plans that work for each patient.

I am excited to share with you some recent developments in the understanding and treatment of IC/BPS. Researchers and clinicians now recognize that this condition is not one-size-fits-all. We now understand that the symptoms of IC/BPS can come from the bladder, outside of the bladder, or even from the brain. To better understand Interstitial Cystitis and Bladder Pain Syndrome, it is necessary to divide patients into smaller subgroups based on their symptoms, history, and clinical findings. This process is called phenotyping and allows for a better understanding of the causes of IC/BPS, enabling clinicians to tailor treatment plans to each unique individual based on their phenotype(s).

Through this book, I aim to provide hope and help to those suffering from IC/BPS. This novel approach of breaking down the large group of IC/BPS patients into smaller subgroups is a meaningful change in how patients will be treated and ultimately find relief of symptoms. I will describe each phenotype in detail and outline clues to help you determine which phenotype best reflects your history and symptoms. Understanding what phenotype(s) you have will facilitate more targeted treatment. This information will allow you to chart a journey to wellness and symptom relief. Although there is no known cure for IC/BPS patients currently, ongoing focused research on the smaller subgroups or phenotypes provides a beacon of hope for the future. As a doctor that has cared for thousands of IC/BPS patients, I believe that this fresh approach will provide much-needed answers and relief for those struggling with this elusive condition. I hope to help newly diagnosed and long-time sufferers of IC/BPS create a roadmap to better health and well-being.

Chapter 1

How to Use This Book

Welcome to the journey to wellness for patients with Interstitial Cystitis and Bladder Pain Syndrome. In Part I, I will summarize how to diagnose IC/BPS and provide tools to help define symptoms corresponding to subgroups or phenotypes. I will also provide advice that is pertinent to all IC/BPS patients, including lifestyle changes and dietary advice. This will allow patients to make changes now to improve their symptoms. As you start to identify with specific phenotypes, additional, more focused treatment options will be discussed.

In Part II, I will start by looking at the big picture and then zoom in on smaller subgroups or phenotypes by describing their typical characteristics. I will explore individual phenotypes, their potential causes, and common symptoms associated with each phenotype. The hope is that patients will identify with a phenotype that fits their history and symptoms. It is typical to have more than one phenotype, so keep an open mind as I describe each one.

As we zoom in on the characteristics of each phenotype, there may be something that resonates with your history and symptoms. For instance, a patient may have classic bladder symptoms but also have symptoms from pelvic muscles, or there may be other chronic pain conditions present, such as fibromyalgia or irritable bowel syndrome, suggesting a brain-processing phenotype. You should consider all potential phenotypes and therapies to achieve optimal relief of symptoms. I recommend you collaborate with your medical practitioner to develop a care plan that is best for you.

In Part III of this book, I will bring everything together by exploring associated conditions often seen in IC/BPS patients. These associated conditions, such as incontinence, recurrent urinary tract infections, and symptoms related to menopause, need to be addressed to get optimal symptom relief. I will discuss the different treatment options available for each condition, and how they can be integrated into your personalized care plan.

I will also focus on special populations such as men and children and explore the unique challenges IC/BPS presents in these groups. This information is crucial for patients and caregivers to better understand how to manage symptoms in these individuals.

Next, I will discuss how to avoid and treat symptom flare-ups and pain with intimacy. Finally, the roadmaps for patients will summarize the information pertinent to each phenotype, allowing you to create an individualized care plan. I will give case presentations that are representative of each phenotype. *Names have been changed to protect patient privacy. Each patient is unique, and they may need different approaches to achieve optimal symptom relief. The goal is to provide patients with the knowledge and tools needed to manage their symptoms effectively and improve their quality of life.

It is important to note that this book is not intended to provide medical advice, and it is strongly recommended that you consult with a medical practitioner before changing your care plan. Remember, you are the best advocate for your health and well-being, and I hope this book will empower you to take control of your IC/BPS journey.

Finally, in Part IV, I will elaborate on individual therapies, as well as alternative and nontraditional therapies. It is essential to collaborate with your medical practitioner to develop a care plan that identifies the best treatment options for your specific phenotype(s). Your practitioner should also be available to provide guidance and support throughout your treatment journey.

This new way of breaking down IC/BPS may not be known to all clinicians yet, so it is crucial for patients to advocate for themselves and share the information provided in this book with their caregivers. I include references from medical journals to support this process.

As patients navigate their journey to wellness, it is important to remember that knowledge is power, and this is a rapidly evolving time for IC/BPS. The goal of this book is to provide information that will help patients achieve remission from symptoms, with remission lasting for many years. So, let's get started on this journey to wellness together!

Chapter 2

Diagnosing Interstitial Cystitis and Bladder Pain Syndrome

Typical Symptoms of Interstitial Cystitis or Bladder Pain Syndrome.

Patients experiencing Interstitial Cystitis (IC) or Bladder Pain Syndrome (BPS) often report feeling an unpleasant sensation, such as pain, discomfort, or pressure, which is felt to be related to the bladder. Other common urinary symptoms related to the bladder area, such as frequent urination and urgency, may also be present. For many patients, the urge to urinate always seems to be present, and although there may be some relief from the urgency after urination, it is not always the case. Symptoms can vary widely, with some patients experiencing no pain but a constant urge to urinate or pressure, while others experience tremendous pain that may be localized or widespread, radiating into the lower back, vagina, testicles, upper thighs, or elsewhere. Symptoms may wax and wane, with some good days and some unbelievably bad days. Some patients may also experience muscle spasms in the pelvic area, making it difficult to release urine, and may have difficulty starting the flow of urine or experience feelings of incomplete emptying. It is not uncommon for patients to be unable to urinate at all.

IC or BPS can have a significant impact on a patient's quality of life. The symptoms can be distressing and unpredictable, and can lead to anxiety, depression, and social isolation. It is important to remember that you are not alone on this journey. IC/BPS is a complex and heterogeneous condition, and each patient's experience is unique. Some patients may have symptoms that are primarily related to the bladder, while others may have symptoms that originate outside the bladder, such as from the pelvic muscles or nerves. Some patients may have symptoms that are related to the brain's processing of pain signals, which can magnify and exacerbate the sensation of pain. When the brain is involved, there are often other chronic pain conditions present, such as irritable bowel syndrome, fibromyalgia, and vulvodynia, to name a few. Therefore, an accurate diagnosis and personalized treatment plan are crucial for effective management of IC/BPS. Patients should work closely with their healthcare providers to identify their specific phenotype(s) and develop an individualized care plan to achieve optimal symptom relief.

To receive a diagnosis of IC/BPS, patients must experience symptoms for at least six weeks, and clinicians must rule out other conditions that can mimic IC/BPS. The diagnosis of IC/BPS is a diagnosis of exclusion. This can be challenging because several conditions can cause similar symptoms, such as infections, tumors, endometriosis, and neurological conditions, to name a few. As a result, many patients experience delays in diagnosis. Misdiagnoses are also common, with patients sometimes being labeled with recurrent urinary tract infections or chronic prostatitis instead of IC/BPS. Unfortunately, not all primary care clinicians are familiar with the symptoms and presentations of IC/BPS. Therefore, a thorough evaluation by clinicians with an open mind and knowledge of IC/BPS is crucial for a proper diagnosis.

Diagnosis: Initial Evaluation

Careful history, as well as physical examination, makes the initial diagnosis. A review of history for trauma, infections, and past surgeries is all important. A review of current medications and past therapies tried, as well as a history of other diagnoses such as irritable bowel syndrome, fibromyalgia, and neurologic conditions, are all important clues. It is important to note that there is no single test that can definitively diagnose IC/BPS, and the diagnosis is often made through a combination of the patient's history, physical examination, and the exclusion of other conditions that can cause similar symptoms. A multidisciplinary approach involving urologists, gynecologists, urogynecologists, physical therapists, and pain specialists may be necessary for proper diagnosis and management of IC/BPS.

Bladder Diary

A bladder diary is a simple and effective tool for patients to track their urinary habits and provides valuable information for healthcare providers. By recording fluid intake, urination frequency, and urine volume, patients can gain insight into their bladder function and help identify potential underlying causes for their symptoms. Healthcare providers can use bladder diaries to monitor the effectiveness of treatments and can adjust therapy as necessary. It is recommended that patients complete a bladder diary at least once, and, ideally, periodically, throughout their treatment journey.

How to do a bladder diary

1. Get a notebook or use the bladder diary provided at the end of the book (Toolbox).
2. Record the date and time you start the diary.
3. Record everything you drink during the day, including water, juice, milk, etc., along with the quantity consumed.
4. Record every time you urinate during the day and night,

including the time, volume, and any symptoms you experience, such as urgency, leakage, or pain.

5. Use an old measuring cup or a "hat" that fits under the toilet seat to measure the volume of urine passed. Your clinician may be able to provide one for you, or you can find one online as a "urine collection hat."

6. Repeat this process for a minimum of 24 hours, and ideally three days, to get an accurate picture of your bladder function.

When completing the bladder diary, it is essential to be as accurate as possible. Record everything you drink and urinate. It's also important to be consistent in the measurement of urine volume, using either ounces or cc. Thirty cc equal one ounce.

After completing the bladder diary for several days, you can use the information to determine your average bladder capacity and frequency of urination. To calculate your average bladder capacity, take the total volume that you urinated and divide by the number of times that you went. For example: 600 cc urinated, divided by 10 times, would be an average bladder capacity of 60 cc. It is helpful to break this down into average bladder capacity when awake vs. average bladder capacity when sleeping. The bladder capacity may also help with identifying which phenotype best fits with your symptoms.

A normal bladder can hold 8-10 ounces (about one cup) before you start feeling a mild urge to urinate, and around 12-15 ounces (about 1.5-2 cups) when it is full. We tend to hold a larger volume at night when asleep, so bladder volumes are typically larger at night.

A bladder diary provides valuable information about how the bladder functions. It helps to determine the maximum volume of urine that can be comfortably held during the day and if this volume is normal at night. It can also show if treatment is increasing the bladder capacity and reducing daytime and/or nighttime frequency. The diary will help quantify the improvements that have been made over time, even if they are subtle.

You can download a free workbook and journal that includes a copy of the bladder diary at https://icjourneytowellness.com or by scanning the following QR code.

Cystoscopy

There are specific diagnostic tests that can aid in the diagnosis of IC. One such test is cystoscopy, which involves the insertion of a flexible or rigid tube with a camera into the urethra and up into the bladder. This allows the doctor to look at the bladder and urethra visually and check for signs of inflammation or other abnormalities. Clinicians often do cystoscopy to rule out other causes for bladder symptoms.

While IC/BPS is usually not visible on an office cystoscopy, the doctor is looking for other conditions that can mimic IC/BPS, such as endometriosis on the bladder, prostatic issues, tumors, stones, and foreign objects left from previous pelvic surgery, such as sutures or mesh. It is important to exclude other potential causes of symptoms before making a diagnosis of IC/BPS. Cystoscopy is necessary to rule out other conditions when blood is seen on urinalysis. Clinicians may also perform cystoscopy to look for Hunner's ulcers or lesions in the bladder.

Some IC/BPS patients have microscopic blood in their urine, with no other cause found. Some IC/BPS patients have ulcers, in which case we can see Ulcerative Interstitial Cystitis on a simple office cystoscopy.

While cystoscopy is not necessary to make the diagnosis of IC/BPS, it can reveal ulcers or Hunner's lesions from IC.

An ulcer or Hunner's lesion shows up as a red spot, like someone has poked you in the eye. Sometimes there is an actual ulcer or crater in the center of the lesion. There may be one ulcer, or there may be multiple. Hunner's ulcers are more prevalent as you get older, and some doctors will consider a cystoscopy if you are over fifty years old, or if you have a strong smoking history. A history of smoking is clearly linked to an increased risk of bladder cancer, and cystoscopy allows a look at the bladder to rule this out. If there is a history of endometriosis, this can also implant on the bladder, causing symptoms like IC/BPS, so cystoscopy may be considered in those patients. There have been some studies that have found an increased prevalence of ulcers in men. My experience has shown this as well. The doctor that is evaluating you will consider your symptoms, exam findings, risk factors, age, urinalysis, etc. and decide if cystoscopy is recommended or not.

Cystoscopy and hydrodistension

Some patients will have a cystoscopy under anesthesia, and in this scenario, we can fill the bladder fuller than what is tolerable in an office setting. The act of distending or stretching the bladder is called hydrodistension. Hydrodistension allows for a measurement of the capacity of the bladder under anesthesia. When cystoscopy is done under anesthesia, Hunner's ulcers or lesions or any other abnormal areas can be biopsied if needed.

Hydrodistension is not required to make the diagnosis of IC/BPS. In the past, doctors performed hydrodistension to look for glomerulations, or small hemorrhages, that were felt to be a hallmark of IC/BPS. There is now evidence that normal asymptomatic patients may show glomerulations, and patients that have the symptoms of IC/BPS may have no glomerulations. Studies have shown no link between the severity of symptoms and the number of glomerulations seen with a hydrodistension.[1]

As with any surgery involving anesthesia, there are risks, though small. Some patients will feel temporarily worse for a few weeks after a hydrodistension. Many patients find hydrodistension can be therapeutic, with an improvement in symptoms. In a recent literature review, 60 percent or more patients had an improvement in symptoms at six months.[2] I have had several patients find hydrodistension therapeutic for their symptoms and repeat the distension every year or two based on their symptoms. Everyone is different.

Urodynamics

Patients who experience frequency and pain may sometimes have other symptoms related to their nervous system, such as numbness in their legs or back problems. They may experience significant urinary difficulties, such as slow urinary flow, difficulty emptying the bladder completely, or significant leakage. In these cases, we may perform an additional test called urodynamics to better understand the function of the bladder muscles and nerves. This test can help provide more information about the bladder's ability to hold and release urine. It is important to note that urodynamic testing is not typically needed for the diagnosis of IC/BPS but may be considered in certain cases to provide a more comprehensive evaluation, especially if there are problems with emptying the bladder or with incontinence.

Urodynamic testing is a diagnostic test clinicians perform in the office. During this test, the patient urinates on a special commode to measure the urine flow rate or how fast the urine comes out. After that, a small catheter is placed into the bladder to measure the volume of urine that remains, and the bladder is refilled while the pressure

---

1   Wennevik GE, Meijlink JM, Hanno P, Nordling J: The role of glomerulations in bladder pain syndrome: a review. J Urol 2016; 195: 19-25.

2   Clemens JC, Erickson DR, Varela NP, and Lai HH: Diagnosis and treatment of interstitial cystitis/bladder pain syndrome. J Urol 2022; 208: 34-42.

inside is recorded. Additional sensors can record pelvic muscles as well. This test helps the doctor to understand if there are bladder spasms, muscle issues, or nerve problems. It will also help determine why there is incontinence or difficulty emptying the bladder.

Although urodynamics is unnecessary for the diagnosis of IC/BPS, it can be extremely helpful if other symptoms of bladder dysfunction are present. Since each person's symptoms are unique, tests may be required to determine what is happening. Your clinician will recommend testing based on your specific medical history, symptoms, and physical examination findings.

Questionnaires

There are several validated questionnaires that can help track your symptoms and response to therapy. There are also questionnaires that can screen for symptoms of prolapse, central sensitization syndrome, or voiding dysfunction. I have included several here. These questionnaires are not used to diagnose IC/BPS but can help to measure current symptoms and the impact those symptoms are having on your quality of life. It is helpful to do the questionnaires at the beginning of your journey, and later to assess improvements made with therapy. Some of these questionnaires are available in the toolbox at the end of the book. You can also access the links to the questionnaires at http://icjourneytowellness.com or by scanning the QR code below.

Questionnaires:
- **Interstitial Cystitis Symptom Index (ICSI)/Interstitial Cystitis Problem Index (ICPI)**: Also known as the O'Leary-Sant IC Questionnaire. This questionnaire is appropriate for men and women. It measures urinary and pain symptoms and assesses how problematic symptoms are for patients with Interstitial Cystitis.[3]

  This is an excellent questionnaire to use to help track your symptoms. Record your scores and then reassess after a few months to see if the score has lowered, indicating improvement.
- **Pain Urgency Frequency (PUF) Questionnaire:** This is an eight-question survey, appropriate for men and women, that assesses urinary and sexual function, as well as pain response.[4]

  This questionnaire, developed by C. Lowell Parsons, MD, is useful in screening patients with chronic pelvic pain. Not only does the survey assess symptoms, but it also measures how bothersome those symptoms are. Scores range from 0-35, and the questionnaire only takes five minutes to complete. A score greater than 12-13 should suggest consideration of a diagnosis of IC/BPS. The score for those with a diagnosis of IC/BPS can be followed to assess symptoms over time.
- **Queensland Female Pelvic Floor Questionnaire**: This survey is appropriate for women and assesses pelvic function. Subsections assess bladder function, bowel function, prolapse symptoms, and sexual function.[5]
- **International Prostate Symptom Score (IPSS):** The AUA symptom index was developed to help assess for obstruction in

3 O'Leary MP, Sant GR, Fowler FJ Jr., Whitmore KE, Spolarich-Kroll J: The interstitial cystitis symptom index and problem index. Urology 1997 May; 49(5A Suppl): 58-63.

4 Parsons CL, Dell J, Stanford EJ, et al: Increased prevalence of interstitial cystitis: previously unrecognized urologic and gynecologic cases identified using a new symptom questionnaire and intravesical potassium sensitivity. Urology 2002 Oct; 60(4): 573-8.

5 Baessler K, O'Neill SM, Maher CF, et al: A validated self-administered female pelvic floor questionnaire. Int Urogynecol J. 2010 Feb; 21(2): 163-72.

men. It has seven questions covering frequency, nocturia, weak urinary stream, hesitancy, intermittent urination, incomplete emptying, and urgency.[6]

The IPSS uses the AUA symptom index and has been adopted internationally as the tool to help screen for lower urinary tract symptoms that can indicate obstruction. The IPSS includes a quality-of-life question that helps to indicate how bothersome the urinary symptoms are to you. We also use this questionnaire in women that have symptoms of obstruction or a slow stream. If you have symptoms of obstruction, the IPSS score can be followed to check for progression of symptoms or improvement. Symptoms are mild if the score is seven or less, moderate if the score is 8-19, and symptoms are severe if the score is 20-35.

- **National Institutes of Health (NIH) Female Genitourinary Pain Index (F-GUPI)**: Questionnaire for women that assesses IC/BPS symptoms, severity, and impact on quality of life. This is a modification of the NIH Chronic Prostatitis Symptom Index, adjusted for women.[7]

  This is another tool to monitor symptoms over time.

- **National Institute of Health (NIH) Male Genitourinary Pain Index (M-GUPI)**: Questionnaire for men that assesses pain, urinary symptoms, and quality-of-life impact of chronic prostatitis/IC/BPS. This tool for men with pelvic pain can be used to measure symptoms over time.

- **Central Sensitization Inventory**: This inventory is appropriate for men and women and is used to assess for symptoms of central sensitization syndrome and for other chronic pain

---

6 Barry MJ, Fowler FJ Jr, O'Leary MP, et al: The American Urological Association symptom index for benign prostatic hyperplasia. J Urol. 1992 Nov; 148(5): 1549-57.

7 Clemens JQ, Calhoun EA, Litwin MS, et al: Urologic pelvic pain collaborative research network. Validation of a modified National Institutes of Health chronic prostatitis symptom index to assess genitourinary pain in both men and women. Urology 2009 Nov; 74(5): 983-7.

conditions that may be seen in the brain-processing phenotype.[8] A score of 40 or higher on part A should raise the question of a diagnosis of central sensitization syndrome.

These questionnaires are useful to measure symptoms and their impact on you and your quality of life. They can give you a score that quantifies the symptoms that you are having. Other questionnaires are useful to screen for symptoms such as urinary obstruction, prolapse, bowel issues, central sensitization, or sexual dysfunction. We often use these questionnaires in clinical trials to assess response to therapy of new treatments.

8   Neblett R, Cohen H, Choi Y, et al: The central sensitization inventory (CSI): establishing clinically significant values for identifying central sensitivity syndromes in an outpatient chronic pain sample. J. Pain 2013 May; 14(5): 438-45.

Chapter 3

Advice for Everyone

Living with a chronic illness like Interstitial Cystitis or Bladder Pain Syndrome can be a challenging journey. When the cause of the disease is not known and there is no known cure, it makes the journey especially difficult. IC/BPS has no visible signs, which means those around you may not understand the extent of your suffering. Even though you do not have outward signs of pain or discomfort, it does not mean you are not suffering silently. This can take a toll on you emotionally and physically in many ways. It may lead to problems at work and in relationships if those around you do not really understand what you are dealing with. Your bladder and pelvic pain may not be a topic you want to discuss with coworkers, so where does that leave you? There are many things that you can do as you navigate life with IC/BPS. By focusing on self-care and seeking support from others who understand what you are going through, you can improve your quality of life and gain control of your future.

Support and physiological quieting.

If you have been diagnosed with IC/BPS, realize that you are not alone. Millions of people around the world are also living with this condition. Consider joining a local or online support group to help connect with others who understand what you are going through. Just knowing that you are not alone helps. Many support groups also offer resources for partners or family members of individuals with IC/BPS.

Living with a chronic illness can be physically and emotionally draining, and it is easy to feel overwhelmed or stressed. Lack of sleep can contribute to increased stress levels and cortisol levels, which can worsen your symptoms. By reducing stress and finding time for self-care, you can improve your overall well-being and better manage your symptoms.

When dealing with stress and pain, techniques that quiet the nervous system can be helpful in reducing symptoms of anxiety and nerve overstimulation. There are several ways to practice physiological quieting, such as deep breathing, meditation, mindfulness exercises, yoga, tai chi, stretching, and gentle aerobic exercise. Spending time in nature can also have a positive effect on our well-being, so consider a walk in the park. Look at the flowers, trees, and birds around you. Sometimes just a warm bath and calming music can help you relax and quiet the nervous system. Many of our smartphones and smartwatches have a simple breathing app. Try it! By incorporating these simple techniques into your daily routine, you can reduce stress, have a positive effect on your overall well-being, and better manage IC/BPS symptoms. Remember that self-care is an important part of managing a chronic illness. Prioritizing your mental and emotional health can make a significant difference in your quality of life.

Avoid straining with urination or bowel movements.

To manage IC/BPS symptoms, it is important to avoid constipation or straining to urinate or move your bowels. Adequate hydration and having fiber in your diet is a good place to start. When you limit your fluid intake, it not only causes the urine to become concentrated and more irritating to the bladder, but it can also contribute to constipation.

We need water and foods high in fiber to have stool that is not like little rabbit pellets or, worse, like concrete! Water is your friend.

It is a good habit to relax when you sit down to urinate or move your bowels. There is a natural tendency for the pelvic muscles to tighten when you walk around all day holding your urine, and this becomes worse if you have urgency or pain. The pelvic muscles need to relax to allow the urine and the stool to come out.

When you sit to urinate or move your bowels, the first step is to relax. Sit comfortably on the toilet. Do not perch on the edge or hover over the seat. Men sometimes find it is easier to relax the pelvic muscles when sitting to urinate. Some people have found that elevating the feet slightly puts you in a better position for relaxation of the pelvic floor. A stool to rest your feet on or a Squatty Potty® works wonders if you have difficulty with constipation or have a slow stream.

Consciously try to relax the pelvic muscles when you are on the toilet. Try to visualize the pelvic floor dropping into the basement. One technique that helps the pelvic floor to relax is to put your hand on your lower abdomen; as you breathe in, focus on your hand rising, and you will feel the pelvic muscles dropping down. Take a deep breath and blow out slowly, like blowing out a birthday candle. This will allow the urine to flow with less stress on the bladder. This breathing technique will make it easier to move your bowels as well.

Hydration

Diet and hydration play a critical role in managing IC/BPS symptoms. As the saying goes, "We are what we eat and drink." The bladder, especially if very inflamed or if in a flare, will be especially sensitive to the urine. One common mistake that many IC/BPS patients make is limiting fluid intake due to frequent urination. Unfortunately, limiting fluid intake can have negative consequences.

When you do not drink enough fluids, urine becomes very concentrated and is irritating to the bladder wall. Hydration is critical to keep urine diluted and help reduce irritation. If you do not drink enough fluids, then there is not enough water to dissolve minerals and other substances in the urine, which can lead to crystal formation. These crystals can form kidney stones. The crystals are also felt to cause burning with urination and burning or pain on the labia or vulva. No one wants to be urinating what feels like sand!

Drinking more fluids is also crucial to preventing urinary tract infections. My mantra to patients has always been, "Dilution is the solution to pollution!" By increasing fluid intake, the bladder is rinsed more frequently, preventing bacteria from sticking to the lining of the bladder and potentially causing infection. Hydration also helps to rinse out waste products that can irritate the bladder and helps to prevent crystal formation.

Remember, everyone benefits from hydration. Everyone is different, and the amount of fluid you need in a day varies based on your activity. If you live or work in a hot environment, or if you have chronic diarrhea, you may need more fluids. You can overdo it, so if your urine is very dark, drink more water. If it looks clear like water, you may be overdoing it. Usually, if you feel thirsty, that is a good clue you need to increase your fluid intake. Unfortunately, there are some medications that cause dry mouth, making it harder to tell if you are thirsty, or just dry. It is usually better to drink smaller quantities throughout the day, rather than a large amount at once.

Reducing stress

Anything that you can do to help reduce stress is beneficial. No matter what your phenotype, whether you have IC with ulcers or Bladder Pain Syndrome, stress has a way of sneaking into our lives. Stress will stimulate the sympathetic nervous system, increase pain, frequency, and muscle spasms, and have a negative impact on your overall well-being.

Do not be afraid to talk to your boss about modifications to the workspace that may help lower your stress. Ask for a stand-up desk if you feel sitting all day bothers you. Speak to your family and get the support you need to help reduce your stress levels. The key here is to speak up and not be afraid to ask for what you need.

With the COVID pandemic, the ability to work from home has been an enormous help for many patients. No more long stressful commutes, worrying about where to find a bathroom. You can wear nice, loose, cozy pants and have ready access to all your tools that help you keep your symptoms at a minimum. Pain psychologists can address past or present life stressors and help provide coping strategies. Do not be afraid to ask for help and be willing to accept it when offered. No one gets a medal for toughing it out.

Advocate for yourself.

You know better than anyone what you are feeling and whether the treatment plan you have is helping. Obviously, if you are not following the plan, then you may not be getting the relief you need. If you are experiencing side effects or lack of improvement from a medication or treatment, do not just stop it or change the dosage without consulting with your provider. Serious side effects can occur if you change the dosage or use medications prescribed for others. If your provider is not knowledgeable in IC/BPS, then try to find a provider that is.

The Interstitial Cystitis Association and the IC Network are both excellent resources to help find a healthcare provider in your area that treats IC/BPS. Seek out local support groups or online support groups for more information about IC/BPS and for the sense of community that they can provide. Remember that what works for one individual will not necessarily work for you. As you have learned, this is a very heterogeneous, mixed group of patients with different phenotypes, and with many varied reasons for symptoms. Try to be patient with yourself. This will help limit the frustration that is typical with this chronic condition.

The American Urological Association (AUA) recommends that the effectiveness of treatments should be assessed periodically, and ineffective treatments should be discontinued. Every treatment decision is a shared decision between you and your provider. You and your provider should outline the risks and benefits and discuss alternatives. In most cases, a multidisciplinary approach to treating IC/BPS works best.

Pain management is an important part of living with IC/BPS. Pain management specialists can help you deal with pain that may limit your daily activities. If you have a plan in place to deal with an IC/BPS flare, then you can act quickly before it gets out of control. Do not be afraid to discuss these concerns with your provider. You are the best advocate for yourself.

Part II

Which Type of Interstitial Cystitis or Bladder Pain Syndrome Do You Have?

In Part II, we will start by breaking down the large group of IC/BPS patients into smaller subgroups. This process is called phenotyping. It allows for a better understanding of the possible causes of IC/BPS and enables clinicians to tailor treatment plans to better suit each unique individual based on their phenotype(s). It is very common to have more than one phenotype, so keep an open mind, consider your clues, and read about all the phenotypes. Each phenotype will be described in detail, and treatments typically used for that phenotype will be discussed. Finally, what we know from research is included at the end of each chapter. It can be shared with your clinician if desired. Appropriate references are included for this purpose.

The large group of IC/BPS patients are divided into three groups. First are phenotypes that arise from the bladder or urethra, the tube that drains the urine. Second are phenotypes that arise from outside the bladder, such as from adjacent muscles or nerves. And third is a phenotype that is associated with the brain and central nervous system called the brain-processing phenotype.

Each of these groups are then divided further, until seven phenotypes in all are described. It is very common for patients to have more than one phenotype, so reading about all of them is recommended. As each phenotype is described, I will provide some clues that may help you identify with that phenotype. This process of identifying your IC/BPS phenotype involves your clinician, so working closely together will help you move forward on your journey.

Chapter 4

Breaking Down IC/BPS Into Smaller Groups

Patients with IC/BPS make up a large, very mixed group, with a variety of reasons for having symptoms. By breaking this large group into smaller groups, it is easier to identify probable causes of symptoms, thus making it easier to find treatments that help ease those symptoms.

The concept of dividing patients into smaller subgroups is not new. In 2007 the European Society for the Study of IC/BPS (ESSIC) proposed a subclassification of different types of IC/BPS. The subgrouping was based on the findings seen on cystoscopy and hydrodistension. The ESSIC classification scores patients based on hydrodistension and biopsy findings of mast cells, fibrosis, and inflammation.[9] This system is still widely used in Europe. Because cystoscopy and hydrodistension with biopsy are not required in the US to diagnose IC/BPS, this system is not used in the US.

In 2009 Dr. J Curtis Nickel from Queens University in Canada, and Dr. Daniel Shoskes from the Cleveland Clinic, described the UPOINT clinical phenotype system. This system described six different domains

---

9   van de Merwe JP, Nordling J, Bouchelouche P, et al: Diagnostic criteria, classification, and nomenclature for painful bladder syndrome/interstitial cystitis: an ESSIC proposal. Eur Urol 2008; 53: 60-7.

or groups of patients, based on symptoms felt to be related to Urinary, Psychosocial, Organ-specific, Infection, Neurologic/systemic, and muscle Tenderness symptoms.[10] The UPOINT system was changed to the INPUT system in 2017 by Crane, Lloyd and Shoskes. They removed the urinary domain and added a domain for patients with ulcers.[11] The UPOINT system is still the phenotyping system that is currently used by the Canadian Urological Association as the foundation for their guidelines for IC/BPS management.

Dr. Christopher Payne has proposed a slightly different phenotyping system that breaks IC/BPS into five groups. The first is Ulcerative Interstitial Cystitis (IC). The other four groups describe patients with no ulcers and are called Bladder Pain Syndrome (BPS). The four Bladder Pain Syndrome groups are the following: bladder-derived phenotype; muscle or myofascial phenotype; neuralgia or nerve phenotype; and the last includes patients felt to have brain-processing issues with multiple pain disorders or central sensitization syndrome.[12]

More recently, Dr. J Curtis Nickel has proposed nine different clinical phenotypes, which may help guide treatment.[13] Using clinical phenotypes has been helpful to guide therapy. As you can see, there are many ways to divide up the large mixed group of IC/BPS patients.

This book attempts to make it easier to understand the phenotypes as clinicians currently envision them. The goal is for you, the patient, to identify with a phenotype, or phenotypes, that best describe your symptoms and history. This focusing in on specific phenotypes provides

---

10   Nickel JC, Shoskes D, Irvine-Bird K: Clinical phenotyping of women with interstitial cystitis/painful bladder syndrome: a key to classification and potentially improved management. J. Urol 2009; 02: 122.

11   Crane A, Lloyd J, Shoskes D: Improving the utility of clinical phenotyping in interstitial cystitis/bladder pain syndrome: from UPOINT to INPUT. J. Urol 2017; 197 (issue 4): 386-387.

12   Payne C: A New Approach to Urologic Chronic Pelvic Pain Syndromes: Applying Oncologic Principles to 'Benign' Conditions. Current Bladder Dysfunct Rep. Topical Collection on Pelvic Pain. March 2015.

13   Nickel JC: Managing interstitial cystitis/bladder pain syndrome in female patients: clinical recipes for success. CUAJ December 2022; 16(12): 393-398.

the basis for developing a more concise treatment plan and speeding up the journey to wellness.

To start, we can break patients down into three basic groups: **Bladder/urethra** as the source of symptoms; **Outside the bladder** as a source of symptoms; and **Brain/Central nervous system** as the source of symptoms. Within each of these three groups, we can describe even smaller groups.

Three possible sources of symptoms in IC/BPS

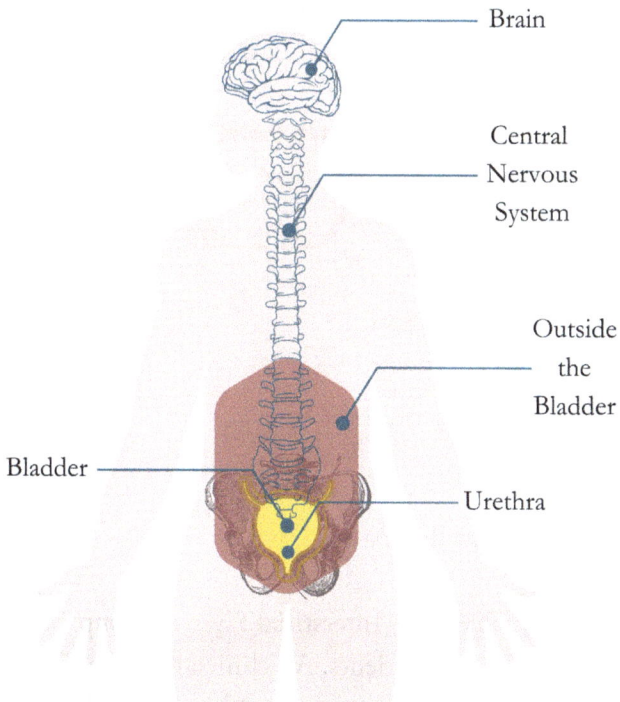

Figure 1: Three sources of symptoms: Brain/Central Nervous System, Outside bladder, and Bladder/Urethra

As the large group of IC/BPS patients are sorted into smaller groups, it is easiest to start by separating out those patients that have ulcers or lesions in the bladder that can be seen on cystoscopy. These lesions are called Hunner's lesions or ulcers. Dr. Hunner first described these lesions in 1918.[14] This group of patients are called **Ulcerative Interstitial Cystitis (IC)**.

Ulcerative Interstitial Cystitis

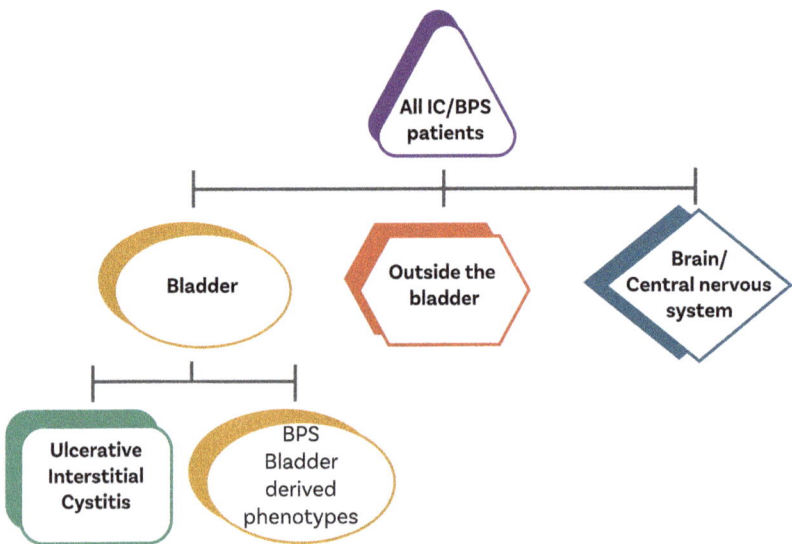

Figure 2: Ulcerative Interstitial Cystitis

Patients with Ulcerative Interstitial Cystitis comprise around 10 to 15 percent of IC/BPS patients. All clinicians agree that Ulcerative Interstitial Cystitis is a disease of the bladder. The bladder looks angry and sore. Clinicians can see these lesions, and, when biopsied, lesions

---

14   Hunner GL: A rare type of bladder ulcer: further notes, with a report of eighteen cases. Journal of the American Medical Association 1918; 70: 203.

will typically show inflammation. This group responds predictably to certain therapeutic measures. But what about everyone else?

Doctors group the remaining 85 to 90 percent of patients into a syndrome called Bladder Pain Syndrome (BPS). A syndrome is not really a disease. The term syndrome is used to describe the combination of symptoms that are seen together. The American Urologic Association defines the symptoms as an unpleasant sensation (pain, discomfort, pressure) that is perceived to be related to the urinary bladder, which may be associated with other lower urinary tract symptoms such as urgency and frequency. Symptoms need to have been present for over six weeks and without evidence of infection or other identifiable causes to explain the symptoms.[15]

It is still common practice for most patients and even clinicians to bundle all IC/BPS patients into the label of "Interstitial Cystitis" or "IC," even though the more accurate terminology is to use Bladder Pain Syndrome if there are no ulcers present. The term IC/BPS includes all patients collectively.

Researchers and clinicians are still developing the description and the subdivision of patients into phenotypes, and more groups may be added soon. There is currently no consensus on how to divide patients with Interstitial Cystitis/Bladder Pain Syndrome (IC/BPS) into phenotypes. This book presents an approach that is a synthesis of current literature and personal experience, which has been advantageous in the 30-plus years of my practice caring for thousands of IC/BPS patients.

While this approach may not be the only way to divide patients into subgroups, it offers a useful starting point for understanding potential causes of symptoms and developing personalized treatment plans. The goal is to improve outcomes for individuals with IC/BPS, and this approach has proven successful in my clinical experience.

---

15   Hanno PM, Burks DA, Clemens JQ, et al: AUA guideline for the diagnosis and treatment of interstitial cystitis/bladder pain syndrome. J. Urol 2011; 185: 2162.

In the following chapters, the three groups—Bladder/Urethra, Outside the bladder, and Brain/Central nervous system—will be evaluated more closely, and individual phenotypes within each group will be described. I will provide clues that will help patients to identify with the individual phenotypes. As I zoom in on the details of each unique phenotype, I will delve into what research has shown us, as well as treatments that have been helpful. By examining the details of each phenotype, we can gain a better understanding of the complex nature of IC/BPS and use this information to develop more individualized and effective treatment plans. The goal is to improve outcomes for individuals with IC/BPS by addressing the unique needs of each subtype or phenotype. The following is a big-picture view of the phenotypes that arise from the Bladder/Urethra, Outside the bladder, and the Brain and Central nervous system. Don't let the chart overwhelm you. As we slowly go through the groups, it will become clearer.

Big Picture of the Seven Phenotypes

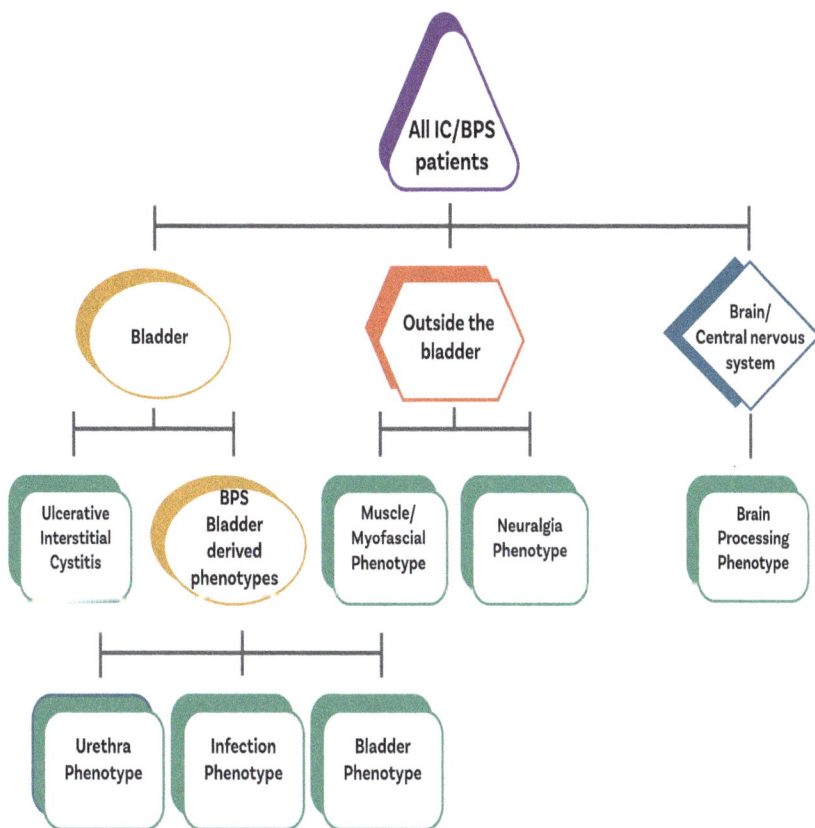

Figure 3: Big picture of the breakdown into Seven phenotypes

Phenotypes arising from the Bladder/Urethra
- Ulcerative Interstitial Cystitis
- Urethral Phenotype
- Infection Phenotype
- Bladder Phenotype

Phenotypes arising from Outside the Bladder
- Muscle/Myofascial Phenotype
- Neuralgia Phenotype

Brain/Central Nervous System Phenotype
- Brain-Processing Phenotype (Multiple Pain Syndromes, Central Sensitization Syndrome)

There are four phenotypes that arise from the bladder or urethra. I will discuss each of these. We will look more closely at the bladder phenotype and consider theories about what might cause symptoms. I have added a breakdown of the bladder phenotype that tries to get to the root cause of symptoms. I have used this to help guide therapy when possible. These are not phenotypes but are possible contributing factors for the bladder phenotype.

The possible contributing factors of mast cell overactivity, nerve upregulation, and an abnormal lining or GAG layer will be discussed in more detail. Understanding what is known from past research can help patients to understand why certain treatments may be tried if a bladder phenotype is suspected. Research is constantly adding clarity to what we know about IC/BPS, and potential new therapies are vigorously being investigated.

Bladder-derived phenotypes have several symptoms in common. Most patients will be sensitive to foods, the acidity of the urine, and high-potassium foods. It is typical to have flare-ups related to certain foods and beverages, as well as seasonal flares, such as in the spring and fall. Frequency of urination both night and day is common. A bladder diary will show that the amount of urine comfortably held in the bladder tends to be less than normal. If you instill an anesthetic into the bladder or into the urethra, symptoms will improve for a short period. If there is no response to an anesthetic trial, it is possible that the symptoms are arising from <u>outside the bladder or urethra</u>.

Next, we will take a closer look at phenotypes linked to structures outside the bladder. These phenotypes involve the pelvic muscles and fascia or tissue surrounding the muscles, and the nerves in the pelvic area. These are the muscle/myofascial and neuralgia phenotypes.

Last, we will look at the brain and central nervous system as a source of symptoms. This group comprises several groups of patients. Patients with multiple chronic pain syndromes and central sensitization syndrome fall into this phenotype. The brain interacts and communicates with the bladder, the muscles, the nerves, and with our environment. It is incredibly complex. The way we perceive the signals sent to the brain varies widely because past experiences influence how we process signals, We will look more closely at possible contributing factors to the brain-processing phenotype.

After all the phenotypes from the bladder to outside the bladder and the brain have been described, the last step will be to piece it all together. It is very typical to have symptoms relating to more than one phenotype.

What has research shown us?

Patients subtyped using the UPOINT phenotyping system, described in 2009 and still used by the Canadian Urologic Association, have been studied. Many patients presented with multiple phenotypes when analyzed with this phenotyping system. Specifically, 12 percent of subjects manifested two phenotypes, 35 percent manifested three phenotypes, 34 percent manifested four phenotypes, 13 percent manifested five phenotypes, and 5 percent manifested all six phenotypes. When specific domains were considered, 96 percent had organ-specific symptoms, and 48 percent fit the tenderness domain, which most closely parallels the muscle/myofascial phenotype. 38 percent of patients fit the infection phenotype, and 34 percent fit the psychosocial domain, which would parallel the brain-processing phenotype.[16]

The UPOINT system differs from what I describe in this book. The key point to take away from the above statistics is that it is quite common to have more than one phenotype. According to some clinicians, over 80 percent of patients with Interstitial Cystitis/Bladder

16 Nickel JC, Shoskes D, Irvine-Bird K: Clinical phenotyping of women with interstitial cystitis/painful bladder syndrome: a key to classification and potentially improved management. J. Urol 2009; 182: 155-160.

Pain Syndrome (IC/BPS) have evidence of muscle issues, such as pelvic floor dysfunction, which contribute to their symptoms. Clinicians commonly refer to this phenotype as the muscle/myofascial phenotype.

By identifying this subtype and addressing the underlying muscle issues, clinicians can develop more effective treatment plans for patients with IC/BPS. This highlights the importance of identifying your phenotype(s) and then developing personalized and targeted approaches to managing your IC/BPS symptoms.

Many times, you may very clearly have the bladder as a source of symptoms and relate to the bladder phenotype. You may also have symptoms of pelvic-floor dysfunction, which is a muscle phenotype. If you have suffered with chronic pain, you may also have upregulation in the brain, which then adds a brain-processing phenotype to the list. You must consider all phenotypes that could be related to your symptoms to experience the best possible relief. So, keep an open mind, and read on.

Chapter 5

Ulcerative Interstitial Cystitis

Ulcerative Interstitial Cystitis (IC) occurs in 10-15 percent of all patients with IC/BPS. Clinicians in the US, Europe, Asia, and Canada all consider this to be a disease of the bladder. All other patients with symptoms of IC/BPS, who do not have ulcers, are called **Bladder Pain Syndrome (BPS).** In this chapter we will explore Ulcerative IC, risk factors, what clues might suggest that you have this phenotype, how it is diagnosed, and finally how to treat it.

Clues that suggest Ulcerative Interstitial Cystitis.

Patients with Ulcerative Interstitial Cystitis typically experience increased frequency of urination both day and night, along with pain. Certain foods may exacerbate urinary symptoms. There may be a tendency to have flare-ups seasonally. Patients with Hunner's lesions will tend to have a more rapid onset of pain and frequency. Bladder capacity when measured is usually lower, and overall symptoms of pain are greater than in other patients with Bladder Pain Syndrome.[17]

Patients with Hunner's lesions also have fewer comorbidities such as

17   Ueda M, Singiku A, Kono J, et al: Low bladder capacity is an important predictor for comorbidity of interstitial cystitis with Hunner's lesion in patients with refractory chronic prostatitis/chronic pelvic pain syndrome. Int. J. Urol 2019; 26 Suppl 1: 53.

fibromyalgia or irritable bowel syndrome, and fewer systemic symptoms or symptoms elsewhere in the body, when compared to patients with no ulcers.

Diagnosis of Ulcerative Interstitial Cystitis.

Ulcerative Interstitial Cystitis patients will have Hunner's lesions or ulcers seen on cystoscopy both in the office and with cystoscopy and hydrodistension under anesthesia. These are red, angry-looking spots on the bladder wall. Picture getting poked in the eye. The big red spot can look remarkably similar. The lesions may have a stellate or star-like appearance with blood vessels radiating out from the center. Some lesions have an ulcer or a crater in the center, with mucus coating it. Lesions may appear whitish. When the bladder distends, the lesions bleed easily, often with a waterfall of blood arising from the lesion. It is common to have multiple ulcers or lesions. Clinicians may biopsy the ulcer or lesion to rule out other causes such as cancer, carcinoma in situ, and other pathology.

Hunner's ulcers or lesions occur more often in older individuals. Men are just as likely to have Hunner's lesions as women.[18] Some studies have found men to be more likely to have ulcers. Ulcerative Interstitial Cystitis is the first of the four phenotypes arising from the bladder or urethra.

18   Lai H, Pickersgill N, Vetter J: Hunner lesion phenotype in interstitial cystitis/bladder pain syndrome: a systematic review and meta-analysis. J. Urol 2020; 204: 518-523.

Ulcerative Interstitial Cystitis

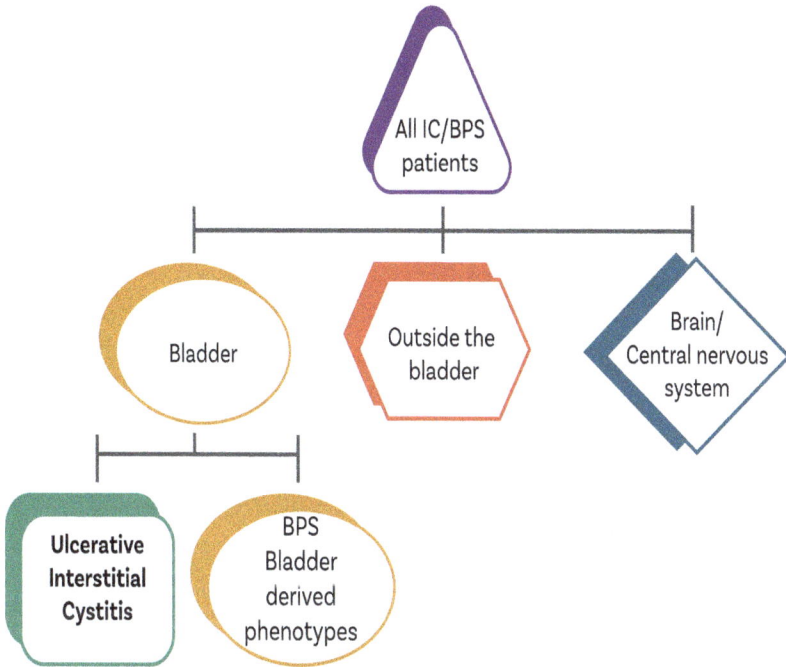

Figure 4: Ulcerative Interstitial Cystitis

What has research shown us?

Being older increases the odds of finding Hunner's ulcers or lesions. Researchers conducted a large observational study of over 1,000 IC/BPS patients from 2009 to 2014, with the enrollment of patients from nine different centers. The MAPP, or Multidisciplinary Approach to the Study of Chronic Pelvic Pain study, has provided significant insight into patients with IC/BPS. The MAPP study observed that Hunner's lesions were increasingly noticed by cystoscopy as the participants aged. They found ulcers in 4 percent of patients under 50 years old, almost 20 percent of patients between ages 50 to 70, and in almost 55 percent of patients over the age of 70.[19]

Researchers have also observed these findings in other studies. The only way to diagnose Ulcerative Interstitial Cystitis is with a cystoscopy, either in the office or under anesthesia. Because the chance of having a Hunner's ulcer is greater with age, it is not unreasonable to have a cystoscopy if you are 50 or older, or if you have been treated for IC/BPS without improvement in symptoms and have never had a cystoscopy. Cystoscopy is also indicated if the diagnosis of IC/BPS is in doubt, or if you have blood in the urine. It is important to know if you have Ulcerative Interstitial Cystitis, as there are specific treatment guidelines for this group of patients. There have been some studies that showed an increased prevalence of ulcers in men, but this has not been shown in other studies. I have seen a higher prevalence of Ulcerative IC in the men in my practice.

Treatment of Ulcerative Interstitial Cystitis.

Diet is important if you have ulcers. Imagine putting vinegar on a canker sore. It burns! Avoiding high-acid foods such as tomatoes or citrus is helpful if you have ulcers. Diluting the urine with good hydration is recommended. Having very concentrated urine will create more symptoms if ulcers are present. Avoiding irritating foods can minimize symptoms and the frequency of flare-ups. The standard lifestyle changes recommended earlier will be helpful as well. Once the ulcers have been treated surgically, bladder retraining may help improve overall bladder capacity, which then helps decrease daytime and nighttime frequency. The toolbox at the end of the book outlines how to do bladder retraining. Additional treatments for Ulcerative Interstitial Cystitis can be divided into medical therapy and surgical therapy.

---

19   Lai HH, Newcomb C, Harte S, et al: Comparison of deep phenotyping features of UCPPS with and without Hunner's lesion: A Mapp-ii research network study. Neurourol. Urodyn 2021; 40(3): 810-818.

Medical therapy for Ulcerative Interstitial Cystitis.

Patients with Ulcerative Interstitial Cystitis tend to feel better if the urine is not overly acidic. Drinking alkaline water, or using a supplement such as Prelief®, an over-the-counter urinary buffer, has been helpful for my patients with ulcers. This is especially important if there is a flare-up.

If a biopsy of the Hunner's lesion shows significant eosinophils or mast cells, I have found adding an antihistamine to be helpful. Antihistamines are available either over the counter or by prescription. An example of a prescription antihistamine would be hydroxyzine. Medications such as gabapentin, or tricyclic antidepressants, such as amitriptyline, may be useful, especially if pain continues to be a significant problem after surgery to treat the ulcers or Hunner's lesions. Intravesical anesthetic cocktails, such as alkalinized lidocaine, have been helpful for patients, especially during a flare-up.

Cyclosporine A is an immunosuppressive agent that is used by clinicians to suppress bladder inflammation. Ulcerative IC patients are more likely to respond to cyclosporine than those with no ulcers. The AUA guidelines give cyclosporine treatment as an option, primarily because of possible side effects from the medication. Doctors should closely monitor patients' blood pressure and kidney function if they are treated with cyclosporine.

Surgery for Ulcerative Interstitial Cystitis.

The American Urological Association (AUA) guidelines outline the current management for patients with Hunner's ulcers.[20] If a patient has a Hunner's ulcer or lesion, it is recommended that they undergo fulguration (with laser or cautery), which burns off the lesion. Many urologists and urogynecologists will do a biopsy to rule out cancer or other pathology at the same time. A biopsy will also show any inflammatory cells in the tissue, which can help guide therapy.

---

20   Clemens JQ, Erickson DR, Varela NP, Lai H: Diagnosis and treatment of Interstitial cystitis/bladder pain syndrome. J. Urol 2022; 208: 34-42.

Besides fulguration, the urologist or urogynecologist can perform an injection with a steroid, such as triamcinolone, directly into the lesion. It is not unusual to require periodic retreatment if symptoms recur.

Several studies have reported significant (75-86 percent) pain relief posttreatment.[21] The improvement of symptoms after treatment has ranged from 2.4 months to 22 months. Each patient is different, and the duration of improvement varies. A choice of either injection of triamcinolone, fulguration, or both may be performed on lesions. An injection with no other treatment saw a 70 percent betterment in symptoms, usually lasting 7-12 months.[22]

I have had patients tolerate periodic steroid injections in the office with local anesthetic, saving them a trip to the OR and general anesthesia.

Neuromodulation is an option for Ulcerative Interstitial Cystitis patients when all other therapies have failed. Some individuals have had outstanding success with this therapy. I will describe neuromodulation in Chapter 24 where treatments are outlined in detail. Substitution cystoplasty (a procedure that enlarges the bladder by adding a patch of bowel), or diversion (redirecting urine to a new reservoir) are options. The surgeon may choose to remove the diseased bladder (cystectomy) or leave it in place. Major surgery should only be a last resort for individuals whose symptoms are obviously coming from the bladder after all other treatments have been tried. The best predictors of success from surgery are end-stage fibrotic or scarred bladder, small capacity under anesthesia, and Hunner's ulcers. Surgery is a weighty decision that should only be considered when all other therapies have been exhausted, and all risks and benefits have been clearly discussed.

---

21   Hillelsohn JH, Rais-Bahrami S, Friedlaner Jl, et al: Fulguration for Hunner's ulcers: Long-term clinical outcomes. J. Urol 2012; 188: 2238.

22   Cox M, Klutke JJ, and Klutke CG: Assessment of patient outcomes following submucosal injection of triamcinolone for treatment of Hunner's ulcer subtype interstitial cystitis. Can. J. Urol 2009; 16: 4536.

Chapter 6

Bladder-Derived Phenotypes
Urethra, Infection and
Bladder Phenotypes

W hen evaluating the bladder as the source of symptoms, first, you have those patients with ulcers seen on cystoscopy, called **Ulcerative Interstitial Cystitis**. We consider all remaining patients to have Bladder Pain Syndrome with a bladder-derived phenotype, as described by Dr. Christopher Payne. Recently, Dr. J Curtis Nickel broke the group down further by adding urethra and infection as distinct phenotypes.[23] As mentioned previously, this is a developing way of trying to separate patients into smaller groups, so that both research and treatments can be more focused.

23   Nickel, JC: Managing interstitial cystitis/bladder pain syndrome in female patients: clinical recipes for success. CUAJ December 2022; 16(12): 393-398.

Phenotypes arising from the Bladder/Urethra

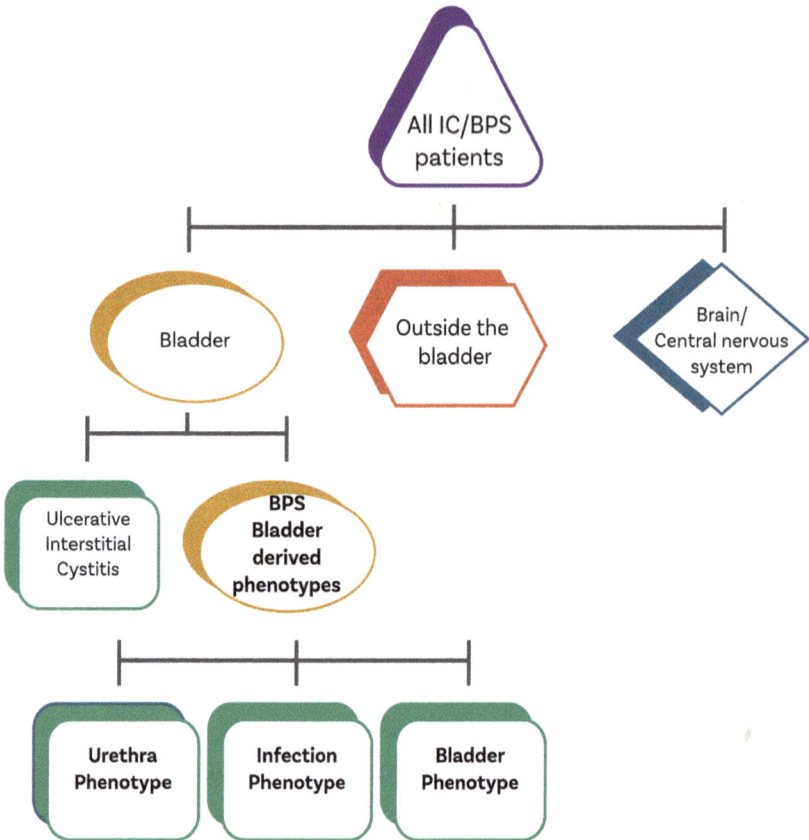

Figure 5: Bladder-derived Phenotypes: Urethra phenotype, Infection phenotype and Bladder Phenotype

Bladder-Derived Phenotypes (Urethra, Infection, Bladder):

The bladder-derived phenotypes make up a large group of patients that are felt to have symptoms arising from the bladder or urethra but without Hunner's ulcers or lesions. These patients will have symptoms primarily focused on the bladder or urethra. It is common to experience a feeling of increasing bladder or pelvic discomfort as the bladder fills. Many patients will experience urgency that can be associated with pain as well. There is usually some relief after urination. The pressure or discomfort triggered by bladder filling usually causes frequent urination both day and night.

Clues that you have one of the bladder-derived phenotypes.

A bladder diary will usually show a smaller-than-normal bladder capacity both day and night. A sensitivity to foods is common, especially acidic or spicy foods. In addition, some will have seasonal flare-ups or seem to be "allergic" to many things. Sometimes hormonal changes will trigger symptoms, as well as stress. It is common to have a flare of symptoms with sexual activity. Patients with the urethral phenotype will have symptoms more focused on the urethra.

If we instill an anesthetic, such as lidocaine, into the bladder or urethra, there will be some relief of symptoms, often only briefly. There will be a little less urgency, or a little less pain. This is a clue that the bladder/urethra is a source of symptoms. If your symptoms are arising from outside the bladder, for example, from the pelvic muscles or nerves, there will be no actual change with anesthetic instillation into the bladder.

There are a multitude of theories as to the cause of bladder inflammation or increased sensitivity to foods or other instigators. Substances like chemotherapy or ketamine might harm the bladder. The bladder may become damaged from extended contact with an excessive amount of caffeine or artificial sweeteners. Radiation can injure the bladder. For patients with the infection phenotype, chronic infections may cause the nerves in the bladder wall to become upregulated and more sensitive. Infection may also cause inflammation in the bladder wall. It is important to remember that even if you have symptoms that seem to arise from the bladder or urethra, other phenotypes such as muscular/myofascial and brain-processing phenotypes may also be present.

Urethral phenotype

Clues that suggest urethral phenotype.

Patients exhibiting the urethral phenotype have signs and symptoms primarily localized to the urethra. Patients will complain of pain, sometimes a sharp pain, and often a burning sensation that is primarily in the urethra or the tube that allows urine to exit the bladder. Other symptoms typically seen with Bladder Pain Syndrome, such as frequency, urgency, and worsening of symptoms during or after intercourse, may also be present. The symptoms in the urethra may be intermittent or constant. Pain may be worse while urinating or may be worse before or after urination.

When the urethra is the primary focus of the symptoms, this group of patients may be treated slightly differently than other bladder-derived phenotype patients. It is important to make sure that there is no pathology in the urethra, such as a stricture or urethral diverticulum. It is necessary to rule out infectious urethritis as a cause of symptoms. If there is evidence of infectious urethritis, doctors may sometimes prescribe a trial of antibiotic based on both history and physical evidence. Urethritis is difficult to diagnose and rarely shows up in a urine culture. Doctors can perform additional tests, but it is not always possible to diagnose an infectious cause. Your provider will use history, risk factors, exam findings, and urinalysis to determine if antibiotics are a reasonable option.

Treatment of urethral phenotype.

If post-menopausal, topical estrogen cream in the area may be beneficial. With menopause, the tissues around the urethra and vagina will become thin or atrophic, and burning or pain can occur. Estrogen cream helps to thicken the tissue, making it less delicate and prone to irritation. Patients should follow the beneficial lifestyle changes outlined earlier. In addition, treatment may include topical medications and oral analgesics such as phenazopyridine or Pyridium®.

For patients with the urethral phenotype, various topical treatments can be helpful. Doctors can prescribe topical lidocaine 2-5 percent gel or ointment for patients with the urethral phenotype to apply as needed to the meatus or opening of the urethra. Post-menopausal patients may benefit from vaginal estrogen. Compounded creams with topical amitriptyline, lidocaine, gabapentin, and baclofen in varying combinations have been helpful for some patients. If muscle tension or spasm is present, topical Valium® is available as a compounded cream. Some patients have found a periurethral block to be helpful. Your medical practitioner will help decide which remedies are suitable for your individual symptoms and history.

We know little about this group of patients. Dr. Nickel did not consider the urethral phenotype a distinct group when he described the initial UPOINT domains in 2009.[24] He added this subgroup in an article, published in December 2022, where he describes recipes for success when treating IC/BPS.[25] This smaller subset is described as a unique phenotype to help guide more focused therapy for the urethral symptoms.

Infection phenotype

Patients with an infection phenotype of Bladder Pain Syndrome have a history of recurrent urinary tract infections. Patients can sometimes continue to experience recurrent infections, which can be mistaken for a flare-up of IC/BPS.

In this group of patients, episodic antibiotic treatment that is appropriate for a positive culture and low-dose antibiotic prophylaxis has been helpful. By effectively managing and treating infections, we can improve outcomes in this group of patients.

---

24   Nickel JC, Shoskes D, Irvine-Bird K: Clinical phenotyping of women with interstitial cystitis/painful bladder syndrome: a key to classification and potentially improved management. J. Urol 2009; 02: 122.

25   Nickel JC. Managing interstitial cystitis/bladder pain syndrome in female patients: Clinical recipes for success. CUAJ December 2022; 16(12): 393-398.

Clues that suggest infection phenotype.

Patients with an infection phenotype have the same symptoms as the bladder phenotype. The major difference is the history of recurrent urinary tract infections. Symptoms of suprapubic pressure or discomfort as the bladder fills are typical, with some relief with voiding. A bladder diary will show lower bladder volumes both day and night. Urgency, a common symptom seen with Bladder Pain Syndrome, may also be present. Patients may continue to have recurrent urinary tract infections, and food sensitivities are common.

What has research shown us?

Studies have suggested that reoccurring infections may cause an upregulation in the nerve endings in the bladder.[26] The nerve endings in the bladder relay signals to the brain that can cause a feeling of urgency, bladder fullness, or even pain. We can consider the nerves in the bladder as a volume control, which has been turned up. Even in the absence of an active infection, the bladder becomes more hypersensitive. As a result, even tiny amounts of urine or bladder irritation becomes amplified and are felt as bladder fullness or significant discomfort or pain. There are additional studies that have found potential links to viruses such as Epstein-Barr that may cause continued inflammation in the bladder wall as well.[27]

Researchers can study the infection phenotype more closely with newer urine testing techniques. It is now possible to do a non-culture, genetic assessment of the urine, which can assess the genetics of bacteria or fungi present in the urine without having to culture them. There is research ongoing to see if this innovative technology will be useful or not in the management of IC/BPS. There has never been a single bacterium or virus that is felt to cause IC/BPS, but now there is evidence

---

26 Koziol JA, Clark DC, Gittes RF: The role of infection in interstitial cystitis/bladder pain syndrome (IC/BPS). Int. J. Clin. Med. and Res 2012; 4(2): 49.

27 Jhang J, Ho H, et al: The role of Epstein-Barr virus infection in bladder of interstitial cystitis/bladder pain syndrome. J. Urol 2018; 199(4S): e512.

that having infections can change the nerves in the bladder wall and contribute to the chronic symptoms many patients have.

Treatment of infection phenotype.

Treatment in this group is like the treatment of the bladder phenotype, with additional focus on preventing future infections. Good hydration and measures to help prevent infections are especially important. Studies have shown that topical estrogen can help post-menopausal women prevent infections. Probiotics may be beneficial in helping prevent infections as well. A discussion with your provider about prophylaxis for intercourse or other high-risk activities that seem to cause infections may be beneficial.

Bladder phenotype

Patients with Bladder Pain Syndrome, who exhibit symptoms arising from the bladder but do not fit into the urethral or infection phenotypes, would be considered to have a bladder phenotype. Many clinicians will lump all three groups together and call them collectively a bladder-derived phenotype.

Clues that suggest bladder phenotype.

The key characteristic of this group is that the symptoms are arising from the bladder. If we place an anesthetic into the bladder, symptoms typically improve, even if just temporarily.

Within this group, there still is a lot of diversity in symptoms, as well as response to different therapies. Researchers have conducted extensive research looking for underlying causes for the symptoms. This research has led to the identification of three potential contributing factors.

The three factors identified are theoretical problems in the bladder that can contribute to bladder symptoms. There is an extensive amount of research that has looked at the bladder as a source of symptoms. In the upcoming chapter, we will explore the potential bladder-related problems that can contribute to symptoms. I have identified certain clues in a patient's history that help to determine potential contributing factors. This approach helps to develop focused treatment plans for each patient. Many patients discover the right treatment only by trial and error. The goal is to be more focused and help patients discover the right treatment quickly, with less trial and error.

Chapter 7

Bladder Phenotype
Potential Contributing Factors and Treatment

In the previous chapter, we discussed patients with a bladder phenotype. This group still has a significant amount of diversity in their symptoms, as well as what treatments will typically help them. There has been extensive research focusing on the bladder and what may contribute to the symptoms of patients with the bladder phenotype. From this research, three key issues involving the bladder have emerged that may contribute to the symptoms experienced by these patients. This chapter will explore these three potential contributing factors.

Researchers have implicated mast cells, a type of immune cell, as a key cause of symptoms for some individuals with the bladder phenotype. Studies have also shown deficiencies in the protective coating of the bladder, known as the glycosaminoglycan (GAG) layer. The third factor potentially contributing to symptoms is an increase in C-fibers or nerve endings in the bladder wall that can cause pain, or an upregulation in those nerves, in essence making the bladder hypersensitive. So just what do we know and how can we use that information to help determine what might work for you?

There have been many studies over the years done to help us understand IC/BPS and theories as to what might cause symptoms. Researchers have recently refuted some theories that clinicians have believed for years. Despite thousands of studies, we still do not know what causes IC/BPS. Studies have identified several key bladder findings that are reproducible and likely interconnected.

I believe that understanding these three key problems and their associated symptoms can help identify which issues may contribute to your symptoms if you have the bladder phenotype. This personalized approach is important because not all medications and treatments will work for everyone. For instance, the source of your symptoms may be attributed to issue one, while the next person may have symptoms originating from the second or third issues. Through pinpointing the factors that are causing your symptoms, clinicians can customize treatment to be specifically designed for you.

As more research unfolds, it may become clear that some of our thoughts about the etiology of the bladder phenotype are wrong. It may be that the GAG layer is not a key problem. As always, keeping an open mind with multidisciplinary collaboration should help us move forward with a better understanding. The following is one perspective of potential problems in the bladder phenotype that I have found useful in developing treatment plans for patients. This is just one way of looking at this subgroup of patients. Other practitioners may have different viewpoints. This highlights the difficulty and challenge of treating patients with IC/BPS, as there is no universal approach for all patients. Each patient's history and examination must be evaluated individually by their clinician to develop an effective treatment plan.

Three potential factors that may contribute to the Bladder Phenotype

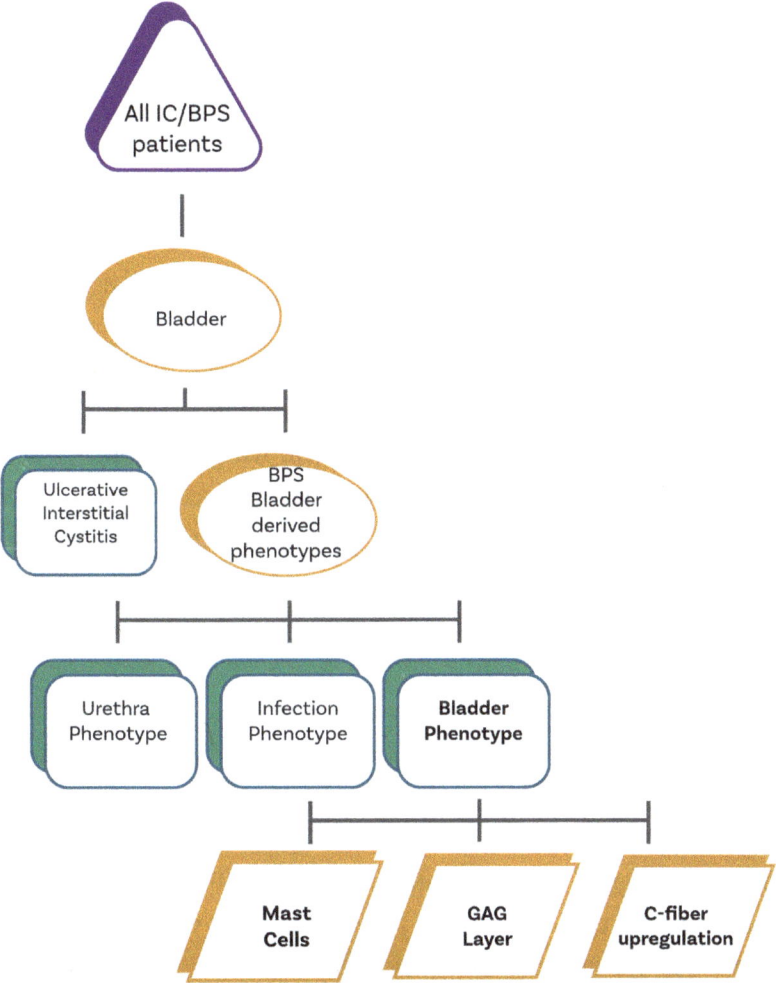

Figure 6: Possible contributing factors in the bladder phenotype

Possible contributing factor number one: Mast Cells

The first key problem associated with the bladder phenotype involves mast cells. Mast cells are part of the immune system. We all have them just like we have red blood cells and white blood cells. Mast cells release histamine in response to different triggers, such as foods, stress, hormonal swings, environmental allergens, and bladder overdistension. The release of histamine can cause the bladder to become inflamed. This inflammation causes the release of cytokines, or molecules that facilitate cell-to-cell communication, which then attracts more inflammatory cells, perpetuating a vicious cycle of more inflammation. There is some evidence that the resulting inflammation from the mast cells may cause the lining of the bladder to become leaky or more permeable, resulting in increased susceptibility to irritants in the urine.

Clues that mast cells may be a contributing problem.

So, what clues would make you think that mast cells are contributing to your symptoms? If you have a history of allergies to multiple environmental factors—medications, foods, soaps etc.—then mast cell activation could be a contributing factor for you. If you are sensitive to and have symptoms from certain foods, then it could be from histamine release from the mast cells. If you notice flare-ups typically in the spring or fall, or during your "allergy" or "hay fever" seasons, then mast cells may contribute to your IC/BPS symptoms. Mast cells can cause cyclical flares because of hormonal changes. There is evidence to suggest that stress can induce mast cell-mediated histamine release. During cystoscopy, if we poke the bladder with the end of the cystoscope, a bright red spot may appear, which may indicate mast cell activation.

What has research shown us?

There have been many studies that have suggested that IC/BPS patients have mast cells as a contributor to symptoms. A few research studies compared the number of mast cells present in bladder biopsies from IC/BPS patients to the amount of mast cells in normal patients by counting them. Some studies have shown more mast cells in IC/BPS patients when compared to normal patients. Other studies have recently refuted this finding. In a study published in 2018, there was no difference in the mast cell counts of Ulcerative Interstitial Cystitis patients when compared to normal controls or patients with chronic cystitis.[28] There is still a lot of research looking at what role the mast cells play in the symptoms of IC/BPS. It may not be the number of mast cells present, but how easily they release histamine and other contents.

If you have more mast cells in the wall of your bladder, then you will have more histamine release in response to your triggers and will have inflammation which then can cause more symptoms. If you have a normal amount of mast cells, but they can be triggered more easily, you will have excessive histamine release. Mast cell stimulation can increase the release of histamine as well as cytokines (aides in cell-to-cell communication), or growth factors that can trigger increased growth of nerve endings.[29] It is the substances released by the mast cells that cause inflammation, which then may cause increased nerve sensitivity and possibly even the leaky bladder lining.

Mast cells are commonly thought of as "allergy cells" by some individuals. If you are highly allergic, it's possible that mast cells are contributing to symptoms. In New England, I have frequently observed IC/BPS patients experiencing increased flare-ups during the spring and fall "allergy" seasons.

Diet will usually play a role if mast cell activation is a contributing factor to IC/BPS symptoms. There are certain foods that are felt to be liberators of histamine. Excessive amounts of these foods could cause an increase in histamine release from the mast cells. The following is a brief list of common foods that will trigger histamine release.

---

28   Akiyama Y, Maeda D, Morikawa T, Niiwi A, et al: Digital quantitative analysis of mast cell infiltration in interstitial cystitis. Neurourol. Urodyn 2018; 37(2): 650-657.

29   Bouchelouche K, Kristensen B, Nordling J, Horn T, et al: Increased urinary leukotriene E4 and eosinophil protein X excretion in patients with IC. J. Urol 2001; 166: 2121-2125.

Foods that can trigger histamine release.

- Bananas
- Tomatoes
- Beans
- Chocolate
- Nuts
- Dairy

Treatments that can help with mast cell overactivation.

There are several medications available that can help stabilize mast cells or act as antihistamines. Over-the-counter cimetidine and antihistamines are commonly used to help those patients with allergy symptoms. Prescription antihistamines such as hydroxyzine can help stabilize mast cells and reduce histamine release. Some of the tricyclic antidepressants, such as amitriptyline, have antihistamine properties. Some patients have found these medications to be beneficial for mast cell activation.[30][31]

Bladder instillations which include anti-inflammatory medications such as a steroid can be helpful for some patients as well. Overall, these are just a few examples of medications that can help stabilize mast cells and reduce histamine.

Possible contributing factor number two: Deficiency in the Glycosaminoglycan (GAG) layer

Problem number two is a deficient or abnormal glycosaminoglycan (GAG) layer in the bladder. The bladder lining is covered with a protective mucous layer like the wax on your car. This coating prevents the urine from touching the bladder wall. If the GAG layer is deficient or leaky, the urine, or components in the urine, can touch the bladder

---

30   Theoharides TC: Hydroxyzine in the treatment of interstitial cystitis. Urol. Clin. North Am 1994; 21: 113.

31   Hanno PM, Buehler J, and Wein AJ: Use of amitriptyline in the treatment of interstitial cystitis. J. Urol 1989; 141: 846.

wall and cause inflammation or irritation. This is like a baby stuck in a wet diaper for a prolonged period, which can lead to skin irritation and inflammation, because of the urine's irritating nature. The GAG layer plays a critical role in protecting the bladder surface from potentially irritating substances in the urine.

Dr. Lowell Parsons did some very eloquent research in the early 1980s, demonstrating that the bladder has a GAG layer and that it can become disrupted or leaky, thus failing to protect the bladder lining from the urine.[32] So, what symptoms may be associated with a leaky GAG layer?

Clues that the GAG layer may be a contributing factor.

Are you overly sensitive to urine contents? Are you sensitive to foods, especially acidic foods, or foods high in potassium, such as bananas, strawberries, or tomatoes? Does Prelief®, an over-the-counter antacid for the urine, help your symptoms? Some Bladder Pain Syndrome patients notice no correlation of their symptoms with diet, so maybe the GAG layer is not the primary problem contributing to symptoms.

Treatments that can help rebuild the GAG layer.

There are certain factors felt to contribute to a healthy GAG layer. One of the early treatments was to instill heparin into the bladder.[33] This was followed by the development of a medication, Elmiron® or pentosan polysulfate sodium (PPS).[34] PPS or Elmiron® is the only FDA-approved oral medication for treatment of IC/BPS and has undergone extensive studies showing its potential to restore the GAG layer. Some recent reports of pigmentary maculopathy, an eye problem that has been diagnosed in patients with long-term usage of Elmiron®, has caused some patients to look at different options.[35]

---

32 Parsons CL, Stauffer C, Schmidt JD: Bladder-surface glycosaminoglycans: an efficient mechanism of environmental adaptation. Science 1980; 208: 605.

33 Parsons CL, Housley T, Schmidt JD, et al: Treatment of interstitial cystitis with intravesical heparin. Br. J. Urol 1994; 73: 504.

34 Parsons CL, Benson G, Childs SJ et al: A quantitatively controlled method to study prospectively interstitial cystitis and demonstrate the efficacy of pentosanpolysulfate. J. Urol 1993; 150: 845.

35 Jain N, Li AL, Yu Y et al: Association of macular disease with long-term use of pentosan polysulfate sodium: Findings from a US cohort. Br. J. Opthalmol 2020; 104: 1093.

Symptoms of pigmentary maculopathy may include difficulty reading, blurred vision, or slowness focusing when going into a dark room. One off-label treatment option is to use Elmiron® as a bladder instillation.[36] Patients that had positive results with the oral medication have sometimes switched over to this option, with less concern about potential vision side effects.

The American Urologic Association has updated the guidelines for treatment of Interstitial Cystitis/Bladder Pain Syndrome to reflect the FDA recommendations from June 2020. It is advised that a thorough ophthalmologic history be obtained before beginning treatment with Elmiron®. Before beginning treatment, we recommend that a preliminary retinal analysis should be performed if a prior eye condition exists. In addition, a follow-up retinal examination six months after starting treatment, and periodically while continuing therapy, is recommended. Everyone must weigh the risks and benefits when considering therapy. Some patients, whose symptoms are improved while taking the drug, have elected to keep taking Elmiron® at the lowest dose that keeps them symptom-free while being observed for any eye changes.

Bladder instillations that might help to restore the GAG layer are heparin instillations, Elmiron® instillations (off-label use), chondroitin sulfate, and Cystistat®. Cystistat® or hyaluronic acid is available in Canada and Europe. Hyaluronic acid is a component of the glycosaminoglycan or GAG layer. Clinicians can instill these medications into the bladder with a small catheter.[37]

Personally, I like the idea of giving our body the building blocks needed to build or repair the GAG layer and have recommended supplements that have some evidence of doing this. Some of these supplements are

36   Davis EL, El Khoudary SR, Talbot EO, et al: Safety and efficacy of the use of intravesical and oral pentosan polysulfate sodium for interstitial cystitis: A randomized double-blind clinical trial. J. Urol 2008; 179: 177.

37   Morales A, Emerson L, Nickel JC, Lundie M: Intravesical hyaluronic acid in the treatment of refractory interstitial cystitis. J. Urol 1996; 156: 45-48.

Cysta Q®, CystoProtek®, and Cysto Renew® to name a few.[38] There have been studies confirming efficacy for some patients with minor side effects.[39] The key ingredients in these supplements are hyaluronic acid, quercetin, chondroitin sulfate, and other anti-inflammatory ingredients.

Aloe vera, from Desert Harvest, has been studied as well. Aloe vera contains glycosaminoglycans and may help restore the GAG layer, resulting in a decrease in symptoms. A 2016 survey conducted in partnership with the Interstitial Cystitis Association reported symptom improvement in 92 percent of patients. Sixty-three percent of patients noted substantial improvement in urinary frequency and urgency while 70 percent noted improvement in pelvic pain and burning. There is currently a larger clinical trial underway to validate the value of Desert Harvest's aloe vera for treatment of IC/BPS.

In most cases, I see no downside to trying a supplement if the GAG layer is a possible contributing factor, other than the cost. It is important to take the supplement consistently for at least 3-6 months, as time is needed to rebuild the protective coating of the GAG layer.

Possible contributing factor number three: Proliferation of C-fibers, or nerve upregulation in the bladder

The third factor that may contribute to symptoms in patients with the bladder phenotype involves activation or proliferation of the nerve endings in the bladder. The bladder contains many types of nerve endings. Studies have shown that C-fibers are associated with Interstitial Cystitis and Bladder Pain Syndrome. These are the nerve endings that give us the sensation of discomfort or pain. C-fibers release substance P, causing pain. There is evidence that

---

38   Theoharides TC, Kempurej D, Vakali S, Sand GR: Treatment of refractory interstitial cystitis/painful bladder syndrome with CystoProtek—an oral multi-agent natural supplement. Can. J. Urol 2008; 15(6): 4410-4414.

39   Katske F, Shoskes DA, Poliakin R, Gagliano K, Rajfer J: Treatment of interstitial cystitis with a quercetin supplement. Techniques in Urology 2001; 7(1): 44-46.

some IC/BPS patents have more C-fibers than a normal bladder.[40] There have been studies showing some patients have increased levels of nerve growth factor, which causes the C-fibers to proliferate. As mentioned earlier, mast cells can release growth factors when they are activated, which is an example of how these different contributing factors may interconnect.

We can think of a radio with the volume cranked up too high to describe the effects of an increased number of nerve endings. For patients with IC/BPS, a small amount of urine feels like a very full bladder. Similarly, a dull feeling in a normal bladder may feel like severe pain in a patient with IC/BPS. Too many C-fibers will cause everything to be amplified. If an IC/BPS patient is complaining of severe pain as a key component of their symptom complex, it could be a problem with their C-fibers. This could be because of an increased number of C-fibers, or hypersensitivity of the nerve endings in some patients. Severe pain can also be associated with brain hypersensitivity which will be covered when we get to the brain-processing phenotype.

Clues that C-fiber activation may be a contributing factor.

If you experience excessive C-fiber firing or upregulation of the nerve endings, you may have several symptoms. These include more pain or discomfort than normal. What may have been just a nagging urge to urinate seems to be more discomfort or actual pain that can be so severe it brings tears to your eyes. This pain may radiate to the lower back, inner thighs, vulva, testicles, or elsewhere. You may get relief with analgesics or anesthetic instillations that numb up the nerves.

Most patients that have nerve upregulation as a contributing factor to their symptoms will feel pain as the bladder fills and will have some relief after they urinate. If an anesthetic agent such as lidocaine is instilled into the bladder, numbing it up, there should be some relief of the pain for a brief time while the anesthesia is working. Most

---

40   Regauer S, Gamper M, Fehr MK, Viereck V: Sensory hyperinnervation distinguishes bladder pain syndrome/ interstitial cystitis from overactive bladder syndrome. J. Urol 2017; 197: 159-166.

patients will see a low volume on their bladder diaries during the day, and often at night as well. Acidic foods and foods high in potassium may be triggers for pain. Think of vinegar touching a canker sore. If the nerve endings are sensitive, acidic urine will tend to cause more pain.

What has research shown us?

Research suggests that constant inflammation in the bladder wall triggers the release of cytokines, which are substances that allow cells to communicate with each other. This can be likened to calling in the army for combat, wherein inflammatory cells, nerve growth factor, and other inflammatory mediators are summoned. As a result, the bladder volume control gets turned up, leading to more symptoms. Research has suggested chronic infections in the bladder can cause upregulation of the nerves, causing symptoms.

This upregulation of the nerves seems to occur gradually. Therefore, those that have experienced IC/BPS symptoms for many years may be more likely to experience severe pain in the bladder. Having IC/BPS for many years does not mean upregulation of the nerve endings in your bladder will occur. Many patients will have other phenotypes arising from outside the bladder as a source of their symptoms. The key is to minimize inflammation early on. It is important to remember that every individual is unique. The aim is to determine the possible contributing factors *you* have, so clinicians can address them in *your* treatment plan.

Treatment options which may help if nerve upregulation is a contributing factor.

You may have observed that activities such as yoga, meditation, or deep breathing, which quiet the nervous system, make you feel a little better. There are many other therapies that can quiet overly sensitive nerves. Oral medications can turn down the volume of the nerves. For instance, medications such as gabapentin or pregabalin can help tone down nerve upregulation. Similarly, tricyclic antidepressants such as amitriptyline are beneficial in reducing nerve oversensitivity.

Oral analgesics, such as phenazopyridine or Pyridium®, are helpful, especially in a flare.

Bladder instillations can be especially useful in numbing the nerve endings, providing relief of symptoms. An anesthetic cocktail that uses alkalinized lidocaine has been highly effective. We teach some patients to catheterize themselves so they can do a daily instillation to wind the nerves down. Other patients opt for weekly or biweekly use of an anesthetic cocktail or use it only if having a flare-up.

There are several complementary treatments that are less well-understood but have been effective, including medical marijuana, acupuncture, TENS units, and other forms of neuromodulation. The intravesical injection of Botox®, a neurotoxin, is currently being studied and shows promising results in reducing symptoms from nerve upregulation in the bladder. With the help of your healthcare provider, you can explore these options and determine which treatment is the best fit for your specific needs.

Because the brain processes the signals from the nerves in the bladder, the constant pain signals can cause hypersensitivity in the brain as well. Some patients may even have nerve hypersensitivity elsewhere in the body.

Chapter 10 will delve into the complex interactions between the brain and the nerve signals it receives in greater detail. If pain makes up a significant part of your symptoms, this chapter will be crucial in understanding how pain signals are processed and what measures can be taken to ease chronic pain.

Chapter 8

Phenotypes Arising from Outside the Bladder

Muscle or Myofascial Phenotype

Next, we will delve into those phenotypes that originate from **outside the bladder.** Most patients in this group present with pelvic-floor muscle disturbances or tenderness. This is classified as the muscle or myofascial phenotype. The second group is smaller and comprises patients that have a neurologic cause for their pain (from nerves outside the bladder) and symptoms of Bladder Pain Syndrome. This group is called a neuralgia phenotype.

Phenotypes Arising from Outside the Bladder: Muscular or Myofascial Phenotype

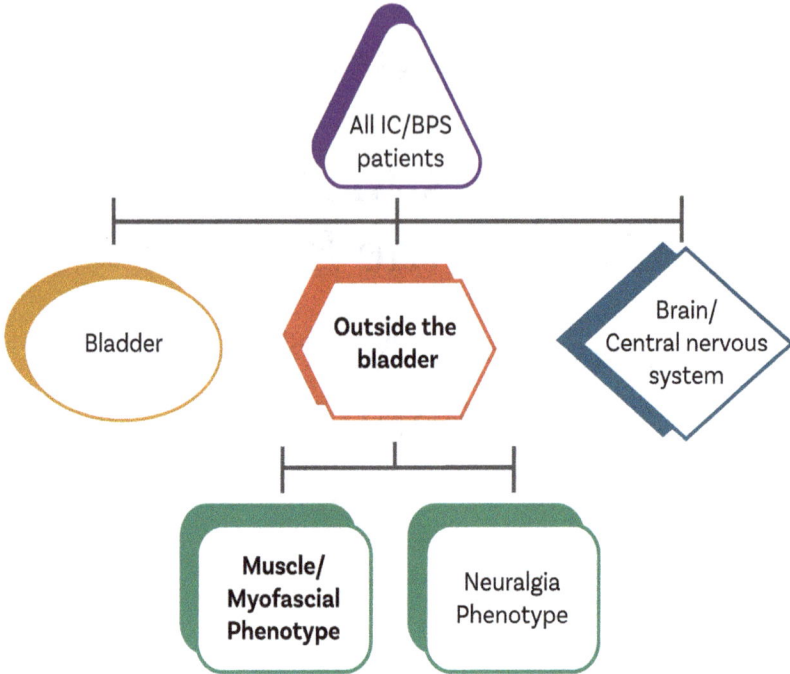

Figure 7: Outside the Bladder as a source of symptoms: <u>Muscle or myofascial phenotype</u>, and Neuralgia phenotype.

Muscle or myofascial phenotype

Many patients will report that their symptoms started after some sort of trauma that may have affected the pelvis. A fall with a fractured tailbone, or even a pelvic fracture, may have preceded Bladder Pain Syndrome symptoms. For some patients, it might have been a difficult delivery that triggered the symptoms or a hysterectomy or other pelvic surgery, which might have created scarring in the surrounding muscles or fascia. The fascia is the tough leathery coating that attaches to the muscles. Some patients seem to get symptoms related to sports or exercise, excessive bike riding or motorcycle riding. Sexual trauma or sexual abuse can be an inciting cause. Patient symptoms are like those with bladder phenotypes, but there are some differences.

Clues that you may have the muscle/myofascial phenotype.

If the pelvic muscles cause your symptoms, you may have muscle spasms that will feel more like a throbbing pain or pressure. Some will describe it as a heaviness, like a bowling ball or a weight in the pelvic area. Pain or pressure may radiate to the vagina, the buttocks, or the rectum. Occasionally, it will feel like low back or even leg pain. If the muscles are spasming, you may have urinary symptoms such as hesitancy when you try to urinate. You may feel you do not empty your bladder all the way. Difficulty with bowel movements is common, even when the stool is of normal consistency. It may feel like a door does not open to allow the urine or stool to pass easily.

On examination, your physician may palpate the muscles and find specific, extremely tender spots we call "trigger points."[41] The pelvic muscles may be tense on examination. Many times, your bladder diary will show frequent urination during the day, but more normal volumes when you are asleep. Often, treatments directed at the bladder will fail. If lidocaine is instilled into the bladder to numb it, you will notice no notable change in how you feel. This is because the pain is originating from <u>outside the bladder.</u>

Scars or bands in the fascia can be a source of myofascial pelvic pain. You can get scarring or nodules in the fascia, as well as in the muscle itself. When touched, these nodules or trigger points will not only cause pain or tenderness but can also reproduce the bladder symptoms of urgency or pressure to urinate. We can inject these trigger points to help ease symptoms, and physical therapy can help with relaxing or massaging the bands and nodules.

---

41   Peters KM, Carrico DJ, Kalinowski SE, et al: Prevalence of pelvic floor dysfunction patients with interstitial cystitis. Urology 2007; 70: 16.

Pelvic floor dysfunction

Researchers and clinicians consider pelvic floor dysfunction (PFD) to be a subset of muscle/myofascial pelvic pain. Clinicians and researchers feel that up to 87 percent of patients with IC/BPS have either muscle/myofascial pain syndrome or pelvic floor dysfunction. Pelvic floor dysfunction (PFD) is the term used to describe a broad constellation of symptoms and/or anatomical changes that are related to abnormal functioning of the pelvic floor muscles. What is usually seen with IC/BPS is a tightening of the pelvic floor or hypertonicity (tenseness) that does not relax when it should, i.e., when you want to urinate or move your bowels. If the bladder must push the urine through a "closed door" because the pelvic floor is not relaxing when you go to urinate, then there is more pressure created in the bladder, and more stress on the bladder.

Clues that you may have pelvic floor dysfunction.

If you have PFD, you may notice a slowing of the stream or a hesitancy that causes you to wait a few seconds to urinate. You may notice your stream stops and starts. Some patients with PFD will have times where they cannot urinate at all and will go into retention, requiring a catheter to drain the urine. Constipation, or difficulty moving your bowels, may bother you, even when the stool is of normal consistency. If you are a female, you may find the vagina is tight. You cannot insert a tampon or have intercourse because of the tightness. Some patients with BPS have pelvic floor problems as the cause of their symptoms.

Other patients may have a bladder or other phenotype as the primary source of their symptoms and develop pelvic floor dysfunction because of bladder pain or constant urgency. It is the "chicken or the egg" dilemma. Is it the bladder symptoms or pelvic pain that cause the muscles to tense up, or is it the muscles that create the bladder symptoms and pelvic pain? I have seen both problems in many of my patients. If there is no history of trauma, and you clearly have a bladder or other phenotype, it is possible you have developed pelvic floor dysfunction secondarily. To get relief from your symptoms, both the primary phenotype and the pelvic floor dysfunction need to be addressed.

Diagnosis of muscle/myofascial phenotype.

To diagnose myofascial pelvic pain or a muscle phenotype with pelvic floor dysfunction, we use a combination of history and physical exam. Do you have hesitancy? How is your urinary flow? Do you have difficulty moving your bowels? Do you feel you are empty? Do you have more frequency during the day and less at night? Do you have specific trigger points? Is there a history of trauma? Typically, patients with primarily a muscle or myofascial phenotype will not notice that foods play a significant role in their symptoms. On examination, your clinician can tell if there is muscle tenderness, spasming, trigger points, or tightness.

You can see the muscle tightness when you use an EMG (electromyogram) with biofeedback or urodynamics. An EMG is a test that is often performed with small electrodes, like an EKG sticker. During biofeedback, we evaluate the pelvic floor when doing exercises, and at rest. With urodynamics, we are recording the muscles of the bladder and urethra to assess for incontinence or difficulty emptying. The EMG will show an elevated resting tone on biofeedback, and similarly, the EMG will show an inappropriate lack of relaxation in the pelvic muscles during urodynamics. You do not need to do these tests to diagnose PFD, but they can objectively show the muscles tightening when they should be relaxing. Urodynamics is done if there is substantial difficulty in urinating, and patients may do biofeedback to help learn to relax the pelvic muscles adequately.

Treatment of muscle/myofascial phenotype.

If we believe you are suffering from myofascial pelvic pain or pelvic floor dysfunction, help is available. If you have evidence of both a bladder phenotype and PFD, you must address both conditions to get relief. If you have PFD that is not treated, then the poor bladder is constantly working harder to push the urine out every time you urinate. The bladder is a muscle that squeezes to push the urine through the urethra. The pelvic floor encircles the urethra, so if it does not relax adequately, you are pushing the urine through a "partially closed door." The bladder must squeeze harder; hence, the muscle works harder. This, just like any muscle, will get bulkier or thicker because of the work it is doing. Think of a weightlifter doing all those bicep curls to get big muscles!

The bladder is like a balloon with a thin elastic wall. You do not want a thickened bladder as it does not stretch as easily as a nice thin bladder wall. Thickening of the bladder wall can lead to urgency and sometimes incontinence or even the inability to urinate at all. So, you can see that it is important for us to address pelvic floor dysfunction, as the effect on the bladder is never good.

We usually employ physical therapy to treat pelvic floor dysfunction and the muscle or myofascial phenotype. Maneuvers to treat pelvic, abdominal and/or hip trigger points, lengthen scarred muscles, and release painful scars are all beneficial. The focus is also on trying to relax the muscles of the pelvic floor and the surrounding muscles that connect to the pelvic floor. In a study comparing myofascial physical therapy to global massage, the PT group had a 57 percent response rate, compared to only 21 percent in the global therapeutic massage group.[42]
You should avoid doing Kegels or muscle-strengthening exercises directed at the pelvic floor. You can learn to relax the pelvic muscles consciously in most cases, but spasming needs to be addressed, and this is best done with a good physical therapist who deals with the pelvic floor.

---

42   FitzGerald MP, Anderson RU, Potts J, Payne C, Peters K, Clemens JQ, et al: Randomized multicenter feasibility trial of myofascial physical therapy for the treatment of urologic chronic pelvic pain syndromes. J. Urol 2013; 189 (Issue 1S): S75-S85.

Doctors sometimes prescribe muscle relaxers. Medications used include things like baclofen, Flexeril®, and other muscle relaxers. I have found intravaginal Valium® for women, and rectal Valium® suppositories in men, to work very well, in combination with PT. Trigger point injections may be beneficial when physical therapy alone does not resolve the trigger points. Neuromodulation with nerve stimulators, such as Interstim® or Axonics®, and Botox® injections into the spasming muscles have been helpful when other therapies have failed.

There may be an increased incidence of PFD in patients with a history of sexual abuse, and this should be taken into consideration when a treatment plan is developed.[43] Researchers estimate that 18-33 percent of patients with IC/BPS have a history of sexual abuse.

Treating PFD and the muscle/myofascial phenotype is truly multidisciplinary, with diet to help avoid constipation, physical therapy, psychotherapy, and urology, gynecology, urogynecology, pain management, and colorectal all involved. The key is to recognize if you have PFD or other myofascial or muscle issues and address whether it is the primary cause of your symptoms or a secondary issue. Either way, it needs to be addressed and treated. Your journey to wellness will not be successful if you ignore the pelvic muscles!

---

43   Peters KM, Kalinowski S, Carrico DJ, Ibrahim JA Diokno AC: Fact or fiction—is abuse prevalent in patients with interstitial cystitis? Results for a community survey and clinic population. J. Urol 2007; 178: 891.

Chapter 9

Phenotypes Arising from Outside the Bladder

Neuralgia Phenotype

When symptoms arise from <u>outside of the bladder</u>, most patients will have the muscle or myofascial phenotype as the source of their symptoms. A smaller group of patients may have pelvic nerve inflammation or irritation as a source of their symptoms. This subgroup, termed the neuralgia phenotype, is the central theme of this chapter.

Neuralgia is a term used to describe pain caused by damaged or irritated nerves. The pudendal nerve is the main nerve of the perineum or the area between the lower buttocks and the genitalia. Think of the area touching a saddle if you were sitting on a horse or a bicycle. The pudendal nerve provides sensation in the saddle area or the lower buttocks, perineum, and the area around the anus and vagina. It is a main nerve in the pelvis that runs from the back of the pelvis to all the muscles in the pelvis and to the skin in the genital area. The pudendal nerve not only provides sensation to this area, but also motor or muscle function to various pelvic muscles. Some patients with abnormal muscles or scarring in the pelvic muscles will also have issues with the pudendal nerve becoming compressed. Thus, the muscle or myofascial phenotype and the neuralgia phenotype may be seen together.

Phenotypes Arising from Outside the Bladder: Neuralgia Phenotype

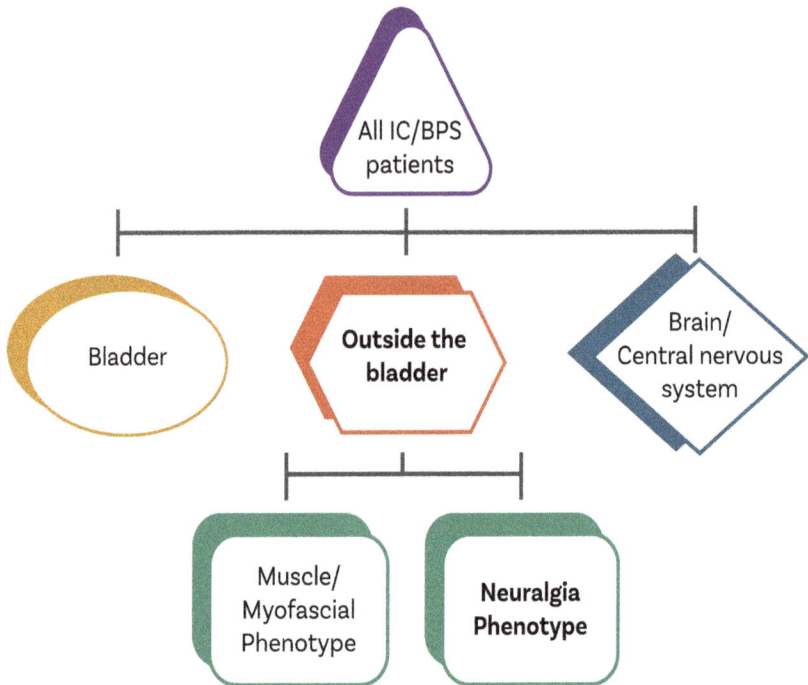

Figure 8: Phenotypes arising from Outside the Bladder: Muscle/ Myofascial phenotype, Neuralgia Phenotype

Neuralgia phenotype: Pudendal neuralgia

Pudendal neuralgia is a long-term pelvic pain that originates from irritation or damage to the pudendal nerve. Symptoms of pudendal neuralgia may include sharp electrical sensations in the pelvis, and sometimes on the skin. You may have shooting pains that go down your leg, like sciatica. Sometimes it will feel like a humming or buzzing feeling. It may feel like a vibration. Many times, it is positional, with less pain if standing but worse if sitting. Sometimes the most comfortable seat in the house is the toilet or sitting on a donut, so patients place no pressure on the perineum. You may feel worse in the evening and better in the morning.

Some people have increased sensitivity, such as pain, when putting on their underwear. Tight pants are uncomfortable. You may feel swollen in the perineal area, like something is in the rectum or vagina. Bowel movements and sex may be painful. Men may notice erectile dysfunction, and there may be difficulty achieving orgasm for both sexes. There can be a general numbness or coldness in the legs, feet, and buttocks. Symptoms may be only on one side of the body or may be on both sides. Some patients have urinary hesitancy, urgency, and frequency. There may be more discomfort *after* urinating, whereas patients with a bladder phenotype will typically feel slight relief after emptying the bladder.

Surrounding muscles or other tissues can often damage or compress the nerve, causing pudendal neuralgia. Hence, the neuralgia phenotype can occur at the same time as the muscle or myofascial phenotype, as one can cause the other. Certain activities that have been associated with pudendal neuralgia are cycling, horseback riding, prolonged sitting, and excessive squatting exercises, to name a few. Fractures in the pelvis or trauma can damage or cause inflammation to the pudendal nerve. Pudendal neuralgia can arise due to complications from pelvic surgery. Trauma from delivering a child has been associated with pudendal neuralgia.

Clues that you may have the neuralgia phenotype.

The typical symptoms of frequency and urgency are present but seem to be less dramatic than in the bladder phenotypes. Pain is a key feature with the neuralgia phenotype. The pain differs from that of the bladder phenotype. Most patients with the bladder as the source of symptoms will find more pressure and urgency as the bladder fills with a sense of relief after the bladder is emptied. With neuralgia, there is typically less relief with emptying the bladder. There may be even more pain when the bladder is empty. The bladder capacity, when measured on a bladder diary, is decreased, but may be closer to normal, and we often see more normal volumes when patients are asleep. Foods will not usually cause worsening symptoms. If we instill an anesthetic into the bladder, there is no notable change in the pain. In addition, the quality of the pain is different. There is less pressure and urgency, and more localized pain, sometimes more to one side than the other. A history of exacerbating activities may be present, either trauma, surgery, or a correlation with excessive bicycling, prolonged sitting, etc. Relief may be obtained by sitting on a donut or padded cushion. Standing may be more comfortable than sitting. These are all clues that you may have a neuralgia phenotype.

Diagnosis of the neuralgia phenotype: Pudendal neuralgia.

Physical examination and history are the key to suspecting that pudendal neuralgia may be at the root of your symptoms. Clinicians will rule out other causes of similar symptoms. On a pelvic or rectal exam, your physician can put pressure directly on the pudendal nerve, which will be very tender and may reproduce your symptoms. An MRI may be useful to help make sure there are no tumors or cysts pressing on the nerve. Occasionally, EMG or electromyography is conducted to evaluate the nerve function. A nerve block can be performed to anesthetize the nerve and assess if the pain is relieved. In the same way that numbing the bladder can reduce the pain originating from the bladder, if the pudendal nerve is the source of the pain, a nerve block with anesthetic will provide temporary relief.

There are some other conditions that may mimic pudendal neuralgia, including sciatica or injury to the sciatic nerve, which causes pain in the lower back. In addition, vulvodynia (pain in the vulva), prostatitis (infection of the prostate gland), and coccydynia (tailbone pain), can all mimic pudendal neuralgia. There are criteria used to help make the diagnosis of pudendal neuralgia, called the Nantes criteria. The criteria for diagnosis are pain in the territory of the pudendal nerve, worsened by sitting, not causing the patient to be woken at night with pain, no objective numbness or sensory loss, and a positive response to a pudendal nerve block.[44]

Treatment of the neuralgia phenotype.

Physical therapy with exercises to relax and stretch muscles that are negatively affecting the pudendal nerve may be helpful. Eliminating causes of inflammation, such as changing your bicycle seat, getting a standing desk, changing your exercise routine, and avoiding constipation, may all be helpful. A TENS (transcutaneous electrical nerve stimulation) machine may be tried to help ease nerve pain. A donut pillow when sitting will usually help, as this eases pressure on the perineum and takes pressure off the pelvic muscles.

Patients have taken drugs such as gabapentin, pregabalin, and amitriptyline to provide relief from nerve pain. Local injections with anesthetics like lidocaine to block nerve pain and with anti-inflammatories like steroids can be helpful in decreasing inflammation of the nerve.

Surgery is an option if all else fails. Decompression of the pudendal nerve is conducted through entrapment surgery, with only a few select centers having surgeons who are qualified to perform the procedure.

---

44 Labatt JJ, et al: Diagnostic criteria for pudendal neuralgia by pudendal nerve entrapment (Nantes Criteria). Neurourol. Urodyn 2008; 27(4): 306-310.

Chapter 10

The Brain and Central Nervous System as a Source of Symptoms

Brain-Processing Phenotype

The brain is an extraordinarily complex organ, as is the central nervous system. All the sensations that we feel go to the brain for processing. How we feel those sensations is determined by the brain. For some, a gentle stroke to the skin can be comparable to a feather brushing the surface, yet for others, the same gentle stroke can be unbearable. If you have ever had shingles, you know how sensations can change. The brain is capable of neuroplasticity and can change and adapt, based on what signals it is receiving, and based on past experiences. A person who has had traumatic experiences may associate certain sensations with a past negative experience, and the brain's response may not be what you would expect. Researchers have revealed that people's perceptions of pain are extremely complicated. We can use neuroplasticity to change the brain in positive ways. This ability of the brain to change is the foundation for cognitive-behavioral therapy and pain reprocessing therapy which can be used to treat the brain-processing phenotype.

In Chapter 7, when the potential causative agents of a bladder phenotype were delved into, the significance of C-fibers and nerve hypersensitivity were discussed. Just as the nerves in the bladder wall can be turned up, or upregulated, the brain and the entire nervous system in the body can get upregulated as well. Comparable to a radio with the volume cranked up, the brain can be hypersensitive, thus intensifying the signals it perceives. Patients with a brain-processing phenotype will have the widespread problem of the brain being hypersensitive to the stimuli or signals it receives. The brain in response may then send excessive signals out to other organ systems in the body. This excessive output of signals from the brain may be at the root of some of the chronic pain disorders seen in this group of patients. This is an area of intense research right now. This ongoing research will help us understand better the complex interrelationship that the brain has with the other systems in the body, as it pertains to pain, and will help guide future treatments for those with chronic pain and overlapping pain disorders.

Brain-Processing Phenotype

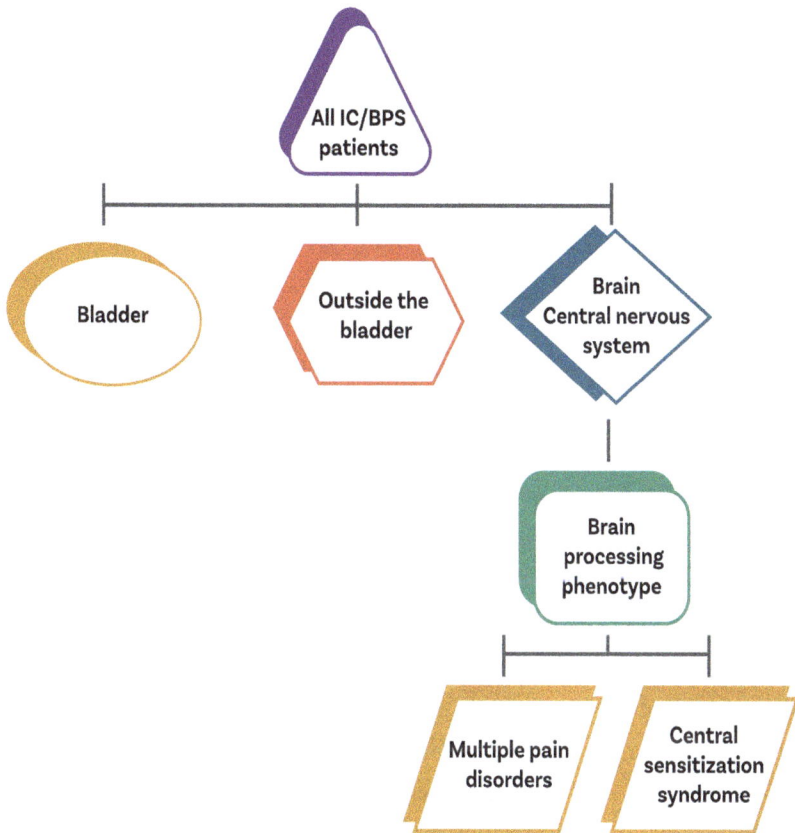

Figure 9: Brain-Processing Phenotype: Multiple Pain Disorders and Central Sensitization Syndrome

Researchers have described at least two separate groups that fall into the brain-processing phenotype. The brain-processing phenotype is divided into two distinct groups: a cohort of individuals with multiple pain disorders and another with central sensitization syndrome. We will discuss these two groups in more detail. There are many other disorders that fall into this group, and how they interconnect with

Bladder Pain Syndrome will become clearer as research in this field advances.

Brain-Processing phenotype: Multiple pain disorders

It has become apparent that patients with chronic pelvic pain often have other chronic overlapping pain conditions. Examples of these chronic pain conditions include irritable bowel syndrome, chronic fatigue syndrome, fibromyalgia, Bladder Pain Syndrome, and vulvodynia.[45] In addition, temporomandibular joint pain and migraines have been shown to be associated.

What has research shown us?

Ongoing research points to the possibility of a central pathogenesis and pathophysiology to these disorders. The NIH-funded Multidisciplinary Approach to the Study of Chronic Pelvic Pain (MAPP) Research Network found that 44 percent of IC/BPS patients had at least one additional coexisting chronic overlapping pain condition. Patients suffering from chronic pain conditions, for example irritable bowel syndrome or fibromyalgia, would be classified as having multiple pain disorders and would be classified as having a brain-processing phenotype. Patients with this phenotype may have other psychological difficulties such as anxiety, depression, or stress either currently or in the past. They may also have a history of early life or adult traumatic events, and often have poor coping skills.[46] There have been studies that have shown that a history of sexual traumatization can cause increased activation of the nervous system, causing hypersensitive brain processing.[47]

---

45   Clauw DJ, Schmidt M, Radulovic D, et al: The relationship between fibromyalgia and interstitial cystitis. J. Psychiatr. Res 1997; 31: 125.

46   Naliboff BD, Stephens AJ, Afari N, et al: Widespread psychosocial difficulties in men and women with urologic chronic pelvic pain syndromes: Case-control findings from the multidisciplinary approach to the study of chronic pelvic pain research network. Urology 2015; 85: 13-19.

47   Sack M, Lahmann C, Jaeger B, and Henningsen P: Trauma prevalence and somatoform symptoms: are there specific somatoform symptoms related to traumatic experiences? J. Nerv. Ment. Dis 2007; 195: 928.

Patients who appear to have chronic overlapping pain conditions seem to have an underlying central nervous system processing disorder. This is not just "in your head." It is a problem in the brain that amplifies pain sensations. A wonderful demonstration of this is phantom pain. Imagine having horrible chronic pain in your foot because of severe trauma. The foot is amputated, but you still feel pain, even with no foot there! The brain is sending pain signals perceived as severe foot pain, even when there is no foot. The brain can send pain signals to the pelvis because of central brain-processing abnormalities, even though there is nothing "wrong" with the bladder. I have had patients with severe IC/BPS that have had their bladder removed because of unrelenting symptoms, only to have the constant feeling of having to urinate, and continued pain persist. But there was no bladder! This was phantom pain. The brain can send signals and give you feelings that are exaggerated, and sometimes falsely perceived. It is important to understand the power and complexity of the brain.

We are learning just how powerful the mind-body connection is. There are a multitude of theories, and ongoing research may help to clarify why this happens. It is common to have multiple phenotypes of Bladder Pain Syndrome. You could have a bladder or muscle phenotype, but also have a brain-processing phenotype.

One study found that one in four patients with chronic pelvic pain related to the urinary tract, either IC/BPS or chronic prostatitis/chronic pelvic pain, had many other complaints outside of the pelvic area. Some of these complaints were pain, such as abdominal pain, and other complaints were things like dizziness, numbness, or palpitations.[48] That study implies that up to 25 percent of patients with other IC/BPS phenotypes may also have a brain-processing phenotype. All phenotypes need to be recognized and treated. Otherwise, there will not be an optimal improvement in symptoms. Additional research studying the

---

48   Lai HH, North CS, Andriole GL, et al: Polysymptomatic, polysyndromic presentation of patients with urological chronic pelvic pain syndrome. J. Urol 2012; 187: 2106.

brain in patients from the MAPP network has demonstrated white-matter abnormalities on imaging.[49] As research continues, we will have a better understanding of the brain-processing phenotype.

Treatment of multiple pain disorders.

The brain-processing phenotype, particularly in patients with multiple pain disorders, is treated by quieting the hypersensitive brain. Physiological quieting, meditation, and mindfulness exercises have been useful in this group of individuals. The goal is to turn the brain down, so it is not sending excessive signals in error. Anything that helps to decrease brain overstimulation is helpful. Noninvasive therapies are recommended, as certain procedures can trigger the brain to respond in a hypersensitive way. An example would be the insertion of a catheter, which may cause an exaggerated response from the brain with more pain, especially if there is a history of past trauma to the genital area.

The focus is therefore on less invasive therapies such as physical therapy and behavioral medicine strategies with a focus on improving coping skills. Cognitive-behavioral therapy and pain reprocessing therapy are examples of psychosocial interventions that have been shown to be beneficial. In addition, medications that focus on decreasing brain hypersensitivity and the central nervous system are helpful. Tricyclic antidepressants, serotonin reuptake inhibitors, and antiseizure medications like gabapentin have been effective for chronic pain patients with multiple pain syndromes. Clinicians have used acupuncture, other alternative therapies, and support groups and found them to be beneficial for some patients. This is an extraordinarily complex problem we are just beginning to understand. An excellent book, *Facing Pelvic Pain, A Guide for Patients and Their Families,* written

---

49   Farmer M, Huang L, Martucci K, et al: Brain white matter abnormalities in female interstitial cystitis/bladder pain syndrome: A MAPP network neuroimaging study. J. Urol 2015; 195: 118-126.

by a multidisciplinary team from Massachusetts General Hospital, is a great resource for patients with multiple pain syndromes.[50]

Brain-Processing phenotype: Central sensitization syndrome

The second group of patients that have a brain-processing phenotype have a condition called central sensitization syndrome. Central sensitization syndrome can be described as a condition in which the central nervous system intensifies sensory input throughout many different organ systems. Patients with central sensitization have hypersensitivity to stimuli that are not usually painful. Examples would be the touch of clothing on your skin, cold temperatures, bright lights, noises, or smells.

This condition was first described back in 1933 and has two primary characteristics: allodynia and hyperalgesia. Allodynia refers to pain that you feel from things that should not be painful. Hyperalgesia refers to an amplified perception of a mildly painful stimulus. We all have receptors in our bodies that will respond to harmful stimuli like extreme temperature or pressure, alerting the brain to the danger that exists. Picture the response you have when you touch a hot stove. With central sensitization syndrome, that part of our nervous system is hypersensitive. As the body reacts over and over to these perceived danger signals, the brain trains itself to recognize these triggers as pain triggers. Simple stimuli, such as touch, pressure, vibration, movement, temperature, smells, etc. all become hypersensitive.

---

50   De E, Stern TA: Facing Pelvic Pain: A Guide for Patients, and Their Families. Massachusetts General Hospital Psychiatry Academy; 2021.

Clues that you may have central sensitization syndrome.

Central sensitization disorders are usually chronic; however, symptoms can wax and wane. Similarly, symptoms may be mild and much more severe at other times. Typical symptoms include the following:

- Headaches
- Abdominal or pelvic pain
- Widespread pain throughout the body
- Poor sleep and fatigue
- Sensitivity to odors, lights, sounds
- Emotional distress like anxiety and depression
- Poor short-term memory and concentration

We know that patients with central sensitization syndrome have physical changes within the nervous system, but the reason is still not clear. It is possible for some that a specific event like an injury, illness, infection, or emotional trauma triggered the changes and the subsequent pain. But sometimes there is no clear-cut inciting cause. Some patients with central sensitization syndrome have a history of family members that are also overly sensitive to their environment. The central sensitization inventory, available in the toolbox at the end of the book, is a questionnaire that will help determine if central sensitization syndrome may be contributing to your pain.

There appear to be some factors that can predispose someone to developing central sensitization syndrome. There is a potential genetic tendency to have a low threshold of pain. A prior history of depression or psychological or physical trauma are predisposing factors. A preexisting anxiety about pain can be a predisposing condition. Researchers have long known that strokes and spinal cord injuries can cause central sensitization syndrome. There are even some theories that recurrent bladder infections can cause central sensitization.[51]

In some patients with IC/BPS, sensations in the bladder are perceived in a hypersensitive way, as is the brain's response to those sensations. Patients with central sensitization syndrome can also have an upregulation in the bladder nerves, like those patients with the bladder phenotype, who have C-fiber upregulation. A few ounces will make the patient feel like they have a full bladder, and mild bladder discomfort will be intensified and felt as pain.

Treatment for central sensitization syndrome.

Several treatments can help ease the symptoms associated with central sensitization syndrome. Most of these therapies target the central nervous system or the associated inflammation that results from central sensitization. Gentle aerobic exercise and other physiological quieting activities have been helpful. Healthy lifestyle habits, including diet, stopping smoking, and avoidance of chemical triggers, are all recommended. Mindfulness, meditation, and the use of visualization techniques have been helpful.

Because there is usually a sensitivity to chemical and environmental stimuli, the home needs to be modified to avoid chemical cleaners, noises, stress, or other stimuli that the body is hypersensitive to. Living in a noisy, busy city is difficult for some patients with central sensitization syndrome, whereas a natural, quiet environment is more comfortable. Nonsteroidal anti-inflammatory medications such as ibuprofen or naproxen have been helpful in treating inflammation. Cognitive-behavioral therapy, pain reprocessing therapy, and other behavioral interventions are immensely helpful as well.

A multidisciplinary approach is the key to dealing with all patients that have central sensitization syndrome as the cause of their brain-processing phenotype. Other psychological therapies, such as

---

51   Cohn J, Brown E, Guo Y, Kowalik C: The relationship between the urinary microbiome and central sensitization in women with overactive bladder. J. Urol 2017; Issue 4S: e398-99.

biofeedback, coping skills, and hypnotherapy, have been useful as well. The key is a multidisciplinary approach to this complex problem. Research is ongoing and provides hope for additional therapies for this phenotype in the future.

Part III

Information to Help Guide You on Your Journey to Wellness

In the next section, we will cover special populations, which include men with IC/BPS and children. In this section, we will also cover conditions that are often associated with IC/BPS or that can sidetrack your journey. These associated conditions are quite common, and must be recognized and treated, especially if they are preventing you from getting optimal relief from symptoms. There are sections on diet and preventing and treating flares, as well as dealing with pain associated with intimacy or sex. Finally, roadmaps for each phenotype will be presented so you can put all the information you have learned into your own personalized wellness plan.

Chapter 11

Demographics and Special Populations

Interstitial Cystitis and Bladder Pain Syndrome affect men and women of all racial and ethnic backgrounds and ages. IC/BPS has been felt to be more common in women than men. Unfortunately, it is often underdiagnosed in men. The median age of diagnosis of IC/BPS is 42-46 years, but the range is wide, with children being diagnosed as well as older adults.

Early prevalence research suggested that 1-5 out of every 100,000 women have IC/BPS, but updated epidemiologic research suggests that many more women may have early symptoms of IC/BPS. Berry et al. in 2011 evaluated the prevalence of IC/BPS using a questionnaire in adult females in the US. [52] The prevalence estimates in women were 2.7-6.53 percent. It would suggest a prevalence of 3.3 to 7.9 million US women aged 18 or older have IC/BPS. Just under 10 percent of these women that had symptoms that met the definition of BPS had been given an IC/BPS diagnosis. This shows that those diagnosed with

---

52 Berry SH, Elliott MN, Suttorp M, et al: Prevalence of symptoms of bladder pain syndrome/interstitial cystitis among adult females in the United States. J. Urol 2011; 186: 540.

IC/BPS are just the tip of the iceberg. Doctors have yet to diagnose many more patients out there with symptoms.

Men with IC/BPS

Men are a special population within the IC/BPS group. We often misdiagnose this group with chronic prostatitis or with other prostate issues. The key difference between frequency and urgency from prostatic issues or chronic prostatitis are the symptoms. If you have frequency and urgency not associated with pain or discomfort in the bladder or suprapubic area, it is not as likely to be IC/BPS. Chronic prostatitis or chronic pelvic pain syndrome (CP/CPPS) patients will have bladder symptoms of frequency and urgency but will have discomfort more localized to the prostatic area or the perineum (area between anus and scrotum). Men with IC/BPS will have the same bladder symptoms of urgency and frequency but will note the pain or pressure to be more localized to the suprapubic or bladder area. Pain with ejaculation is common as well. Men may not be as willing to discuss symptoms of pain, but this clue is important to helping to diagnose IC/BPS, versus CP/CPPS or other prostatic conditions.

In a comparison of baseline symptoms in men and women in the MAPP research group of patients, women had more bladder-focused symptoms compared to men. The most bothersome single symptom for men was pain in the suprapubic or bladder area (34 percent), compared to women (58 percent). In addition, the mean age for men was 46.8 years and in women was 40.5 years of age.[53]

There is some evidence that Hunner's ulcers are more common in men with IC/BPS. Other studies have found the prevalence of ulcers to be similar in men and women.[54] Some would argue that

---

53 Clemens JQ, Clauw DJ, Kreder K, Kruger JN, et al: Comparison of baseline urologic symptoms in men and women in the MAPP research cohort. J Urol 2015; 193(5): 1554-1558.

54 Lai H, Pickersgill N, Vetter J: Hunner's lesion phenotype in interstitial cystitis/bladder pain syndrome: A systematic review and meta-analysis. J. Urol 2020; 204: 518-523.

you should consider cystoscopy in this group because of the possible higher prevalence of Hunner's ulcers. As we have discussed, if you have a Hunner's ulcer or lesion, there are different treatment options, such as fulguration and/or steroid injection, that can significantly help the symptoms. Urologists that treat IC/BPS will assess symptoms, urinalysis, and history to decide if cystoscopy is needed to assist in the evaluation for IC/BPS.

Suskind et al. (2013) assessed the prevalence of IC/BPS and chronic prostatitis/chronic pelvic pain syndrome and found an overlap between the two syndromes.[55] The study showed a prevalence estimate of 2.9-4.2 percent for IC/BPS and a prevalence of 1.8 percent for chronic prostatitis/chronic pelvic pain syndrome. The overlap between the two syndromes was approximately 17 percent. Doctors may label many men as having chronic prostatitis that have IC/BPS. This study suggests that the prevalence in men is closer to that of women than previously thought.

In men with IC/BPS, associated voiding problems can worsen symptoms. Prostatic enlargement or slowing of the stream from obstruction will force the bladder to squeeze harder to urinate. This increased pressure in the bladder can worsen IC/BPS symptoms. Slowing of the stream can be due to pelvic floor dysfunction as well. Evaluation by a urologist will help to determine if there are associated prostatic conditions, or PFD, that can be exacerbating your IC/BPS symptoms.

Children

Children similarly are a special group. Healthcare providers often delay diagnosing IC/BPS in children because IC/BPS isn't considered in the differential diagnosis. Because this is uncommon in children,

---

55   Suskind AM, Berry SH, Ewing BA, et al: The prevalence and overlap of interstitial cystitis/bladder pain syndrome and chronic prostatitis/chronic pelvic pain syndrome in men: Results of the RAND interstitial cystitis epidemiology male study. J. Urol 2013; 189: 141.

many clinicians do not even think of IC/BPS when evaluating children with frequency, urgency, or pain. Treatments useful for adults may not always be an option for children diagnosed with IC/BPS. Many of the medications used in adults are not FDA-approved for children, and similarly invasive procedures would not be tolerated by younger children.

Simple steps like treating constipation and dysfunctional bladder habits can be helpful. Diet is important, especially removing irritants to the bladder. Adding fiber to help avoid constipation and encouraging good hydration is important. Using a stool or Squatty Potty® may help position children for better urination and defecation.

A noninvasive evaluation using an EMG of the pelvic floor (small sticky patches like an EKG) can be done while at rest and with urination, and one can tell if there is evidence of pelvic floor dysfunction. If pelvic floor dysfunction is present, biofeedback and PT for the pelvic floor with dietary modifications would be a good starting point for therapy. Biofeedback can help children with pelvic floor dysfunction learn to relax their pelvic muscles when urinating. Biofeedback is noninvasive, and some centers will have systems that are like a video game, which is engaging for children.

There is not as much literature available on IC/BPS in children. The fundamentals employed for treating adults are similar for children. Try to phenotype the IC/BPS and use the least-invasive treatments first. Keep an open mind and address all phenotypes and associated conditions such as an overactive bladder. The pelvic floor is important, as is the role of the brain. Past traumatic experiences need to be addressed by a qualified pediatric psychologist.

Often, a multidisciplinary approach is necessary, with support from caregivers, educators etc. Often, teachers need to be involved so they understand the need for more frequent bathroom visits etc. Living with IC/BPS as an adult is hard; having it as a child is even harder.

It is important to work with a pediatric urologist with knowledge of IC/BPS in children.

Chapter 12

Role of Diet

There is a lot of discussion about what is a good IC/BPS diet. There is a tremendous amount of variability in individual responses to foods. An individual may have an uncommon response to foods at various times. Whereas you may tolerate certain foods on a 'good' day, you may not tolerate that food on a 'bad' day or when having a flare.

The bladder lining tends to be sensitive to highly acidic urine, to high potassium levels in the urine, and to caffeine and alcohol. On top of this, some people just cannot tolerate certain foods, dyes, and preservatives. Individuals with a muscle/myofascial phenotype, or a neuralgia phenotype, may not notice significant symptom changes with foods.

It is reasonable to not go crazy with caffeine, alcohol, artificial sweeteners, or excessive acid. Patients with an overactive bladder may also find these foods worsen their urgency. I have found that a low-acid diet has been helpful for most patients, and alkalinizing the urine, especially during a flare, seems to help the symptoms. So, what are the foods that IC/BPS patients should try to avoid?

The Top Worst Foods for IC/BPS are the following:
- Tomatoes
- Caffeine
- Citrus
- Very spicy foods
- Diet sodas, especially colas

Other foods that bother some patients are the following:
- Alcoholic drinks
- Chocolate
- Carbonated beverages, including seltzer

The list of foods that have been found to affect patients with IC/BPS is quite long. Not all foods will affect all patients the same way, so how do you know what you can and cannot eat?

The easiest way to find out whether any foods bother your bladder or increase your symptoms is to do an 'elimination diet' for a few weeks. You do this by eliminating all the foods that could be a problem. **The best resources for IC/BPS food lists are the Interstitial Cystitis Association, http://www.ichelp.org, or the IC Network, http://www.ic-network.com.**

If you notice that your bladder symptoms improve while on the elimination diet, then at least one food was contributing to your symptoms. Slowly add back one food at a time. For example, try a few strawberries. If there is no worsening of symptoms after 24 hours, you should be OK. I usually recommend not going crazy with any of the foods. Moderation is the key. After a few days, try another new food. Remember, only one new food every few days. Some patients with IC/BPS become overly paranoid about their diet and will come into the office and report eating only a few foods. I had one patient living on rice and salmon. Clearly not a healthy way of eating. Try to include a variety of fruits and vegetables in your diet. There are good substitution lists available online. It is all about balance.

There are also many good cookbooks available if you are looking for innovative ideas or just need some inspiration from others. I like the idea of a diet that naturally alkalinizes the urine. This involves cutting back on meats and having a more vegetable-centric diet.

You can also help to alkalinize your urine by drinking alkaline water or by using Prelief® supplements, which act to buffer the acid in the urine, especially if you are eating an acidic food such as tomatoes. Some patients will get away with small amounts of acidic foods by taking a Prelief® with that food. It will allow you to expand your diet significantly. Alkalinizing the urine is especially helpful if you are having a flare, or if you have Ulcerative Interstitial Cystitis or a bladder-derived phenotype.

Remember, hydration is important to keep the urine from being too concentrated. Having smaller sips of liquid more often is better for your bladder than chugging a large quantity all at once, which can overload your bladder and create more problems. Remember to have fiber in the diet, as this will help prevent constipation.

Patients that have a problem with mast cells can consider some of the mast cell stabilizing foods.

Mast cell stabilizing foods (good for you):
- Watercress
- Chamomile
- Turmeric
- Thai Ginger
- Apples
- Brazil Nuts
- Peaches
- Onions
- Quercetin-rich Foods (e.g., buckwheat, broccoli, cabbage, asparagus)

Foods that trigger mast cells (bad for you):
- Citrus
- Tomatoes
- Avocados
- Spinach
- Eggplant
- Fermented and processed foods or aged foods
- Gluten-containing grains
- Dairy
- Alcohol

Naturally high histamine foods (bad for you):
- Dried fruits
- Legumes
- Shellfish
- Eggplant
- Spinach
- Avocado

For many patients, histamine and mast cells are not a problem, so these foods may not bother them.

Some patients have tried an alkaline diet, which is more plant-based. If you have lots of allergies, or if you have central sensitization syndrome, you may find that you are extremely sensitive to dyes and additives, or chemicals used in processing or preserving foods. You may be better able to tolerate organic fruits and vegetables and less processed foods. I have had patients try limiting or going gluten-free, and they have found their symptoms improved. A food journal is helpful as you learn how diet affects your symptoms. It is essential to remember that everyone is unique when it comes to diet, and you'll need to experiment to find what works for you. You can download a food journal at https://icjourneytowellness.com or by scanning the QR code.

Chapter 13

Conditions Often Associated with IC/BPS

The confusing part of Interstitial Cystitis/Bladder Pain Syndrome is that we also see it in association with other disorders. It is important to recognize and diagnose these associated conditions, as they may have similar symptoms and can contribute to urinary frequency, urgency, or pain.

Sometimes, the associated conditions can worsen the symptoms of IC/BPS. A good example of this is any condition that tightens up the urinary outlet, making it harder for the urine to flow. If the outlet is obstructed, the bladder will have to work harder and generate more pressure to allow the urine to flow. This obstruction can worsen the IC/BPS symptoms.

Both an overactive bladder and recurrent urinary tract infections are felt to cause an upregulation in nerve endings in the bladder and can cause worsening of IC/BPS symptoms. It is imperative that these associated conditions be recognized and treated. Otherwise, patients will not get optimal relief from their symptoms from treating only the IC/BPS.

We have already discussed overlapping conditions, such as irritable bowel syndrome, fibromyalgia, vulvodynia, and chronic fatigue syndrome. We can see these conditions in the brain-processing phenotype, in patients with multiple pain syndromes. There are other conditions that I have seen commonly overlap with IC/BPS, such as endometriosis, overactive bladder, recurrent urinary tract infections, and voiding dysfunction. We will discuss these associated conditions in more detail.

Endometriosis

There has been a significant overlap seen between endometriosis and IC/BPS as a cause for pelvic pain in women. In one study, 38 percent of the patients who underwent laparoscopy for pelvic pain were diagnosed with IC/BPS.[56] In women who have had a hysterectomy for their pelvic pain, if pain persisted after surgery, IC/BPS was frequently the cause. Many women have come to me with persistent urinary symptoms and pelvic pain after they were treated for their endometriosis. I found them to have IC/BPS in addition to their endometriosis. Both conditions needed to be treated to get symptom relief. Similarly, if you do everything to treat your IC/BPS, but still have cyclical or monthly flare-ups with frequency and pelvic pressure, you may have endometriosis that needs to be addressed as well. A collaborative effort between gynecologists, urogynecologists, and urologists is essential for treating women with chronic pelvic pain.

Vulvodynia/vulvar vestibulitis

Vulvodynia is a chronic pain condition discussed in the previous chapter that outlines the brain-processing phenotype. I find that vulvodynia will often be present in patients with IC/BPS and can be just as debilitating as the IC/BPS bladder symptoms. Vulvodynia

---

56   Clemons JL, Arya LA, Myers DL: Diagnosing interstitial cystitis in women with chronic pelvic pain. Obstet. Gynecol. 2002; 100(2): 337-41.

is a chronic unexplained pain around the opening of the vagina. Several therapies employed to alleviate IC/BPS may be useful in managing vulvodynia symptoms as well. I have collaborated closely with gynecologists that specialize in vulvodynia to optimize the care for these patients. Hydration is important in patients with vulvodynia, as overly concentrated urine or crystal formation will aggravate the condition. Using compounded creams and tricyclic antidepressant medications like amitriptyline or nortriptyline has been useful in the management of vulvodynia. Gynecologists and urogynecologists that specialize in vulvodynia have additional therapies that can be helpful.

Recurrent urinary tract infections

Urinary tract infections can happen to anyone. They occur more often in women than men because of the shorter urethra in women, which allows easier access for bacteria to get into the bladder. There are certain risk factors that increase the chance of getting an infection. Poor hydration is often a contributing factor. I always say, "Dilution is the solution to pollution!" Many patients with IC/BPS limit their fluid intake because of the urgency and frequency that they have. This in turn increases the risk of urinary tract infections.

Another risk factor is menopause and the changes that occur in the vaginal area. Incompletely emptying the bladder can contribute to infections, and we know that many patients with IC/BPS have pelvic floor dysfunction, with occasional difficulty emptying. Men with prostatic enlargement may have incomplete emptying that can increase their risk of infections. Women with prolapse of the bladder, or a cystocele, may not empty completely, increasing their risk of infections.

The last risk factor is having an abnormal bladder lining, which allows bacteria to stick to the surface, rather than rinsing out when you urinate. Patients with ulcers or other areas of inflammation have a lining that can act like VELCRO®, allowing bacteria to adhere to the surface more easily. It is not a surprise that we find urinary tract infections in those with IC/BPS.

Equally frustrating is the fact that a UTI and an IC/BPS flare can have similar symptoms, so patients are never sure of which one they have, a flare or an infection. A simple screen for these situations is to do a urine dipstick test to check for leukocytes and nitrite in the urine. Test strips are readily available online and at the pharmacy. You can find AZO® test strips at most pharmacies. If both nitrite and leukocytes are showing positive, there is a good chance you DO have an infection. It is important to note that if you use over-the-counter AZO® for pain relief (phenazopyridine) or Pyridium®, the urine dipstick may show a positive result for nitrite erroneously. The other difference is that IC/BPS flares do not usually cause burning with urination, but an infection typically will have some burning during or at the end of your stream. If in doubt, it is always best to consult with a health care provider for a urinalysis and/or urine culture.

There are many simple things that can help prevent infections that do not aggravate your IC/BPS. It is always best to start with the simplest things first. Hydration would be the first step and is especially important after activities where bacteria may get into the urethra or bladder more easily. You should urinate after intercourse or intimacy, after swimming or a tub bath, bicycling, exercise, etc.

Cranberry juice can irritate the bladder, but IC/BPS patients usually do well with the supplement D-mannose. D-mannose puts a small particle into the urine which will help stick to bacteria, so that the bacteria do not adhere to your bladder wall as easily. We do not typically recommend this to patients with diabetes. We have found probiotics to help prevent infections in women as well, by improving the bacterial flora around the urethra/vagina. Probiotics are available in both oral and topical formulations. Some patients will use a tiny dose of antibiotics after intimacy or other high-risk activities if that is the trigger for infections. We recommend consultation with your medical provider to determine the best recommendation for you.

If you are post-menopausal, helping to restore the normal vaginal flora or bacteria that naturally live in the vaginal area is helpful. Populating your vagina with beneficial bacteria reduces the room for 'bad' bacterial overgrowth. A topical estrogen cream or suppository can accomplish this, and there are other non-hormonal options, such as hyaluronic acid, which is available as a cream or as a suppository. Revaree®, a hyaluronic acid suppository sold over the counter, is an example of this. A consultation with your medical practitioner will help to determine if you have positive cultures and infection, as well as help to determine the best plan to help you avoid future infections. I have routinely provided patients with a lab slip and specimen cup, so if there is a concern about an infection, a urine culture can be gotten quickly, prior to starting an antibiotic. It is best to avoid unnecessary antibiotic use, as this can cause increased antibiotic resistance as well as vaginitis from killing the good bacteria that live in the vaginal area.

Genitourinary syndrome of menopause

Genitourinary syndrome of menopause or GSM, previously known as vulvovaginal atrophy or atrophic vaginitis, involves symptoms of vaginal dryness, burning, itching, burning with urination, pain with intercourse, urinary frequency, and recurrent urinary tract infections. We can attribute most of these symptoms to the lack of estrogen that characterizes menopause. While these symptoms are usually seen in post-menopausal women, premenopausal women can also experience symptoms.

The reason that symptoms related to menopause are important to treat is because there is a significant overlap with IC/BPS symptoms. Lack of estrogen can contribute to urgency, frequency, and pain during intercourse. It can contribute to burning with urination and urethral pain. Lack of estrogen in the vaginal area can contribute to recurrent urinary tract infections. Sometimes, you will not get optimal relief of symptoms by just treating the IC/BPS, if you ignore the symptoms of genitourinary syndrome of menopause.

We should address bothersome symptoms related to the lack of estrogen in women at the same time as the treatment of IC/BPS. Doctors have used lubricants, moisturizers, and lifestyle changes. Non-hormonal therapy includes nutraceuticals such as phytoestrogen, vaginal laser therapy, and oral ospemifene, which is a selective estrogen receptor modulator. Doctors have also used alternative therapies such as vitamin D, coconut oil, vaginal vitamin E, and probiotics. A variety of hormone therapies, such as estrogens, DHEA, and testosterone, can be administered orally, transdermal, subcutaneously (implant), and vaginally. You have many options available to help ease the symptoms, many of which do not involve estrogen if that is contraindicated for you. If you have symptoms of genitourinary syndrome of menopause and IC/BPS, both need to be treated. You should consult with your clinician to determine the best options for you.

Voiding dysfunction: Obstruction, incontinence, overactive bladder

Besides the typical symptoms of IC/BPS, patients may develop significant urinary dysfunction or urinary abnormalities. It is easier to understand what can go wrong with the urinary tract when you understand how a normal bladder works. The bladder is like a balloon that stores the urine until it is time to urinate. It is made of a muscle that should be relaxed and is elastic, so it can expand to hold the urine without pressure building up. So, we want a nice stretchy balloon, ideally that can hold 10-15 ounces. You do not want to have a balloon made of leather, as it will not stretch to fill with urine, and, if it were to fill, the pressures could be too high, causing problems. Unfortunately, some patients with IC/BPS can develop small, stiff bladders with minimal stretch. Clinicians will call this a fibrotic bladder. Similarly, a bladder that is forced to push the urine through an obstruction will become thickened as the muscles thicken from overwork. The thickened bladder will not stretch as easily and will not hold as much urine. Clinicians call this bladder hypertrophy.

The urethra, or the tube that allows the urine to pass, is surrounded by muscles that help to hold the urine in. When it is time to urinate, the muscles should relax to open the door (sphincter) so the urine can flow out easily. This prevents excessive pressure being generated inside the bladder. Men have prostates that surround the urethra like a donut and, if the prostate enlarges, can cause a narrowing to the tube. Similarly, women can develop prolapse of the bladder into the vagina (cystocele) that, when severe, can cause a kink in the tube, again blocking the door. Both men and women can also develop scar tissue or strictures that can cause a blockage to the urethra.

The bladder and the muscles surrounding the urethra receive signals from the brain to help keep the bladder relaxed when in storage mode and signal the door to stay closed. When it is time to urinate, signals from the brain will tell the door to open, and then the bladder to squeeze so we expel the urine. There are lots of things that can go wrong and cause symptoms of urgency, frequency, leakage, weak stream, or incomplete emptying.

The main urinary difficulties that are seen can be broken down into overactive bladder, urinary incontinence, and outlet obstruction. I will discuss each of these in more detail. Dr. J Curtis Nickel has described this group of patients as an added phenotype of IC/BPS.[57] We commonly seen these problems in the urology practice, and they are not usually associated with pain. I think of this as an associated condition that can be present with any of the IC/BPS phenotypes. The phenotyping of IC/BPS is evolving, and we may ultimately consider this another phenotype, when symptoms are associated with bladder pain.

---

57   Nickel, JC: Managing interstitial cystitis/bladder pain syndrome in female patients: clinical recipes for success. CUAJ December 2022; 16(12): 393-398.

Overactive bladder

Overactive bladder (OAB) is characterized by an urgency that comes on suddenly, often triggered by the sound of running water, stepping out into the cold, or putting the key in the door when you get home. This may be associated with leakage. Patients will have an increase in urinary frequency and getting up at night. You can have urgency with IC/BPS, but it seems to be a more constant or painful urge to void, not a feeling of impending leakage. I will often ask my patients, "If you are stuck in traffic and need to urinate, but you can't, do you have pain, or do you feel you are going to wet your pants?" OAB patients will typically say they feel like they will leak, while IC/BPS patients will be more likely to have increasing discomfort or pain.

If your IC/BPS treatment has significantly improved your pain or pressure, but you still have a lot of urgency, then you may also have OAB. OAB is quite common in patients with IC/BPS. In a recent study of women with IC/BPS, evaluated in the Veteran Affairs Health Care system, of the women with IC/BPS, 79 percent had urinary leakage associated with a strong desire to void.[58]

Overactive bladder is treated in a stepwise fashion, first with behavioral modifications, such as eliminating bladder irritants and exercise. Second-line therapy involves medication that helps to relax an overactive bladder, and third-line therapy involves Botox®, neuromodulation, or PTNS, which stands for posterior tibial nerve stimulation. Using medication to relax the bladder muscle can exacerbate the hesitancy or difficulty emptying that some patients with IC/BPS experience, which can make it poorly tolerated. Medications can also cause dryness and constipation, which can cause difficulty with IC/BPS. I have found PTNS to work well in this group of patients, especially if patients cannot tolerate medication. Botox® is currently FDA-approved for treatment of OAB and is being investigated for

---

58 Dubinskaya A, Tholemeier L, Erickson T, et al: prevalence of urge urinary incontinence among women with interstitial cystitis/bladder pain syndrome. J Urol 2022; 207(supp5): e107.

use in IC/BPS. The risk is retention or inability to empty the bladder after injection. It is important to consult with your medical provider if you suspect that an overactive bladder may be present.

Urinary incontinence

Urinary incontinence is leakage of urine associated with a powerful urge to void, with a cough or lifting something heavy, with bouncing, or even just leakage that happens with no awareness or feeling at all. Leakage can be caused by a bladder muscle problem or be due to problems with the muscles surrounding the bladder or urethra. Leakage may also arise from other structural or neurological problems. Leakage rarely makes the symptoms of IC/BPS worse, but leakage can show that there are other problems that should be investigated. Leakage of urine certainly can affect one's quality of life. It is best to seek consultation with a medical provider that treats urinary incontinence, for evaluation and consultation about treatment options.

Women with stress incontinence, or leakage with coughing, sneezing, etc., may be advised to have surgery for treatment of their stress incontinence. I have had many patients referred to me with worsening of their IC/BPS because of mild obstruction caused by a sling or other incontinence surgery. Conservative therapy is advised if possible, and if surgery is needed, opt for a looser sling, and live with a little stress incontinence, rather than risk worsening the IC/BPS. When the bladder must work harder to push the urine out, the bladder is not happy when you have IC/BPS. Working with a provider with experience treating IC/BPS is important.

Outlet obstruction

When a person urinates, the bladder muscle squeezes or contracts to push the urine through the urethra. If the tube or outlet is blocked because of a mechanical obstruction or the muscles are not relaxing to open the door, the bladder must squeeze harder to expel the urine. This will cause the bladder of a patient with IC/BPS to work harder and will often worsen symptoms of IC/BPS.

Both men and women can have outlet obstruction. We relate the most common cause to pelvic floor dysfunction. When you have a constant urge to urinate or if you have pelvic or bladder pain, the pelvic muscles will tense up to help you "hold" your urine. Unfortunately, when you finally go to urinate, the muscles do not always relax completely, and the door does not open fully. This causes hesitancy, slowing of the urinary stream, and sometimes incomplete emptying. The higher pressures generated by the bladder can cause the bladder muscle to thicken. Now the balloon, which is the bladder, gets thicker as the muscles bulk up, and the bladder does not stretch as easily. Over time, this causes a small bladder and can cause more urgency, incomplete emptying, and sometimes leakage. Outlet obstruction is never good for a patient with IC/BPS.

Pelvic floor dysfunction and the treatment of this has been discussed in the chapter outlining the muscle or myofascial phenotype. We must also address other causes of outlet obstruction. Male prostatic obstruction needs to be investigated and managed, and female prolapse as a cause of obstruction should be considered.

Women can develop prolapse of the bladder, uterus, and rectum because of the weakening of the support structures in the pelvis. Childbirth, menopause, obesity, chronic cough, or lifting are just a few of the risk factors for developing prolapse. If significant prolapse is present, it often feels like a goose egg is coming out of the vagina. Sometimes the bulge or prolapse is visible at the vaginal opening. When the bladder prolapses (cystocele), it can create a kink in the urethra, which can then cause obstruction. If prolapse is suspected, a gynecologist, urogynecologist, or urologist should be consulted for further evaluation. Along with surgical options, conservative therapies are also available.

Men that show signs of obstruction should consult a urologist. There is medical therapy available to help relax the muscles around the urethra to improve the flow of urine, as well as medications to help shrink the prostate. A urologist can do several procedures to help with prostatic obstruction if needed. Once more, we advise you to seek the counsel of a urologist if there are serious indications of slow flow, inadequate evacuation, and hesitation to urinate. The IPSS questionnaire, available in the toolbox at the end of the book, is a good screening tool. A score of eight or above indicates moderate obstructive symptoms, which may be contributing to your IC/BPS symptoms.

Both men and women can develop scar tissue or strictures in the urethra. Infections, trauma, or prior procedures can cause this. Some women develop strictures at the opening of the urethra, related to thinning from menopause. Symptoms of a stricture may be a thin stream or spraying of the urinary stream. If you suspect a stricture, seek the evaluation of a urogynecologist or urologist. Therapy usually involves dilating the narrow-scarred area in the office, and occasionally, the stricture may require surgical intervention to ease the blockage.

Chapter 14

Avoiding and Treating Flares

The dreaded flare is something that all patients with IC/BPS fear. Patients with IC/BPS experience good days and bad days. A flare is a terrible day and sometimes can last a week or longer. Everyone is different when it comes to an IC/BPS flare. If your phenotype is primarily bladder-derived, or if you have Ulcerative Interstitial Cystitis, then the flare may be triggered by foods, stress, allergies, hormones, intimacy, traveling, or allowing the bladder to become overdistended. It is not unusual for there to be seasonal flares during 'hay fever' season. I have had patients that have gone to the dentist and must sit in a chair for dental work for a prolonged period. This caused their bladder to become too full and triggered a flare. Of course, there is always that flare that seems to happen for no rhyme or reason.

The symptoms of a flare will be a worsening of your usual IC/BPS symptoms. Typically, there is more frequency, more pain or pressure, more getting up at night, and that constant feeling like you must urinate. Some will have more urgency to the point of leakage; others may have more hesitancy to the point of not being able to urinate at all. I have had many patients present to the ER with the inability to urinate, only to be catheterized for a few ounces, and then be told there is nothing wrong.

For some, the dull pain that they have been living with is magnified. I have been told that it feels like a "cyanide-soaked tampon," a "hot poker," or that it feels like they are urinating "shards of glass." It hurts! If you have the myofascial phenotype, or a muscle phenotype with pelvic floor dysfunction, you may feel like everything is spasming. Picture a Charlie horse in the pelvis. This will make it hard to move your bowels, urinate, or even move. Lying in bed, curled up with a heating pad, seems to be your only choice.

Patients will often describe muscle spasms like labor pains, a baby's head pushing down on the vagina, or feeling a ball in the vagina, bladder, or rectum. The pressure is intense, and even urinating does not help it. Those with neuralgia will have more electrical shooting pains, with more radiation into the upper thighs or legs. Sometimes there will be sensations of a painful arousal in the clitoral area. Patients with the brain-processing phenotype or with multiple pain disorders may have nausea, vomiting, bowel symptoms, and pain elsewhere in the body. They may feel horrible everywhere. No one wants to have an IC/BPS flare.

Obviously, if you have learned what your triggers are, then you have learned to avoid those triggers. But sometimes flares will happen regardless. Many times, patients will call not sure if what they are feeling is the beginning of a flare, or if it is vaginitis, or a urinary tract infection. Ideally, we try to see them right away to assess the urine and check for vaginitis if the symptoms call for it. But flares seem to happen in the middle of the night and on weekends! So, what do you do?

There are some tools at your disposal. You can get a urine dipstick (i.e., AZO® test strips) at the pharmacy that can help you screen for a UTI. Remember, if you have taken Pyridium® or AZO® for pain relief, the dipstick may show a false positive for nitrites. The strip will tell you if you have nitrites (a byproduct of bacteria), or leukocytes, which are white blood cells, seen with infection. We typically give our patients lab slips to have on hand, so that they can go to the lab for a urinalysis and urine culture if it is not clear if it is a flare versus a true UTI.

Bladder phenotype or Ulcerative IC flare

If you have a bladder phenotype or Ulcerative IC, then I have found making the urine alkaline and coating the bladder with an analgesic is often the best starting point. You can get pH paper to evaluate your urine pH online. Ideally, if you are having a flare, I like to get the pH to 7 or 7.5. You do not want acidic urine, which would have a pH of 5. Drinking alkaline water or using a supplement such as Prelief® or taking a TUMS® may be helpful if the urine pH is very acidic. There are many urinary analgesics out there. Over the counter, you can use AZO® for maximum pain relief, which is phenazopyridine. There are prescription analgesics that we use as well. Some are a combination of medications, which include low-dose methenamine (urinary disinfectant), hyoscyamine (mild muscle relaxer for the bladder), phenyl salicylate (anti-inflammatory), and methylene blue or phenazopyridine. I like these for most patients because they cover several causes of pain. Obviously, if you are having difficulty in emptying, we would not recommend this, as the hyoscyamine could make it harder to urinate. Your provider will counsel you on the best analgesic based on your history, allergies, etc.

Some patients that have used bladder instillations with success in the past will come in for a bladder instillation. The combination of an anesthetic agent, an anti-inflammatory and sometimes sodium bicarbonate as an antacid will get things under control. It is important to dilute the urine, which helps to prevent it from being overly concentrated, so hydration is important. Many individuals will find heat or cold helps. Try to relax. Use all your physiological quieting tricks to prevent the brain from sending more pain signals and an overflow of sympathetic nervous system signals. Most IC/BPS patients have their primary provider on speed dial to help in diagnosing a flare early, so treatment can start quickly. You should consult with your clinician, as having a plan in place will help to reduce some of your anxiety about having a flare.

Infection phenotype flare

The same advice given above would pertain to a flare if you fall into the infection phenotype. Adequate hydration, anesthetic cocktails, and bladder analgesics are all helpful. Urinalysis and urine culture would be indicated if there is any concern that this could be a urinary tract infection. Antibiotic use is based on the urine culture results and the recommendations of your clinician. Because there is evidence of C-fiber hypersensitivity associated with chronic infections, medications that turn down the nerve endings can be helpful if pain is a primary complaint.

Urethra phenotype flare

Patients with the urethra phenotype will receive help from the same treatments as the bladder phenotype. Medical professionals may recommend warm tub baths or soaking to help with the symptoms focused on the urethra. Topical analgesics such as lidocaine gel or ointment may be helpful. Intravesical instillations may help with symptoms, especially anesthetic cocktails. Compounded creams with lidocaine, amitriptyline, gabapentin, and baclofen have been helpful. Valium® suppositories may help if spasm is present.

Muscle/Myofascial phenotype flare

If you seem to fall into the muscle or myofascial phenotype, then relaxation of the muscles is paramount. You can use heat to relax the muscles, and we often administer medications to aid in muscle relaxation. Here is where I will have patients try low-dose baclofen, Flexeril® (cyclobenzaprine), or another muscle relaxer of choice. A vaginal or rectal Valium® suppository can be especially useful to help relax the pelvic muscles. Stretching is helpful, focusing on diaphragmatic breathing, and visualizing the pelvic muscles dropping into the basement. A nice warm bath and anything that you have found that quiets and helps the muscles to relax is also helpful. Some patients have found that chamomile or peppermint tea can soothe muscles and aid in relaxation. There may be some antispasmodic properties from peppermint tea.

Oral analgesics such as NSAIDs, i.e., ibuprofen or naproxen, can be helpful, as can acetaminophen. Remember to always follow the label, as too much acetaminophen is toxic to the liver, and too much ibuprofen or naproxen can damage the kidneys. Even over-the-counter medications can be contraindicated if you are on blood thinners or have underlying kidney or liver problems. It is best to consult with your provider to determine the best medication plan for you. Doctors may prescribe stronger pain medications to patients, which they often use short-term, intermittently when they have a flare. Do not raid your cupboards and start taking whatever you have, as some medications cannot be mixed, and never take a higher dose of medications than prescribed without consulting your provider. Serious side effects and even overdose can occur.

Neuralgia phenotype flare

Patients with the neuralgia phenotype will benefit from the techniques of physiological quieting, such as breathing, guided imagery, stretching, and heat. Patients may find relief with topical anesthetics, like a lidocaine patch. If TENS units have helped in the past, that may be another option. You may be able to soothe muscle spasms associated with the flare with the application of heat and muscle relaxants. Analgesics such as acetaminophen, ibuprofen and naproxen can be used, and clinicians may prescribe stronger analgesics depending on the symptoms. Typical treatments focused on the bladder will not be as helpful unless you also have a bladder-derived phenotype. As always consultation with your healthcare provider is advised to determine the best options for you.

Brain-processing phenotype: Multiple pain disorders/ central sensitization syndrome flare

Oral bladder analgesics and alkalinization of the urine may be helpful, especially in those patients with central sensitization syndrome, as the bladder nerves are often upregulated as well. Instillations of anesthetic into the bladder can provide pain relief when the bladder is affected, and you have had success with anesthetic cocktails previously. The use of physiological quieting techniques outlined previously can help quiet the hypersensitive nervous system. Breathing exercises, meditation, guided imagery, stretching or anything that you have found helps to calm the nervous system should be tried. You need to get your brain to not focus on the signals it is receiving from the bladder, so try to distract it.

Patients with systemic or significant symptoms outside of the bladder will need targeted therapy based on their symptoms, for example, antinausea medications for vomiting, or medications for IBS flare or diarrhea. Patients with a history of trauma or abuse may have flashbacks and severe anxiety, or an exaggerated pain response that occasionally requires a multidisciplinary approach based on their history. A provider that understands your history will guide you both physically and emotionally through a flare. Having a plan in place is helpful before anxiety sets in and things snowball out of control.

The best thing to remember about flares is that they will subside. If you learn your flares are seasonal, often, I will have patients start on an over-the-counter antihistamine to prevent the flare. Journaling can be a helpful technique to improve mindfulness and start honing in on what your triggers are. Everyone is different, and you will learn what works best for you. If you have flares, then knowing that there is a plan in place will help you act quickly when symptoms start. Collaborating with your provider is important, as each patient is different.

Chapter 15

Pain with Intimacy or Sex

Dealing with pain during intimacy can be incredibly challenging for patients with Interstitial Cystitis and Bladder Pain Syndrome. Past painful experiences or flares that have been triggered by intimacy will create anxiety about future interactions, perpetuating the problem. There are several reasons that pain can occur. It may be the bladder that is causing the pain, or it may be the muscles or even the vaginal tissue that is causing the pain. By using the phenotyping process, it is possible to focus on the source of painful symptoms and develop a targeted plan to manage or prevent pain.

Preparing for intimacy can be an enjoyable experience for both partners. Both partners can try doing physiological quieting exercises together. This could involve taking a warm bath and doing some deep breathing exercises with the visualization of a favorite place that you both have enjoyed. Another option is to sit facing each other, with legs dropped to the side in a butterfly position, which can stretch the pelvic muscles, and induce relaxation and quieting of the nervous system. Warm massages of the back, abdomen, thighs, and genitalia can be an intimate form of foreplay that also helps relax the pelvic muscles and calm the nervous system.

Experiencing pain during intercourse or intimacy can be caused by a range of factors. For those with a bladder-derived phenotype or Ulcerative IC, the bladder can be tender and sensitive to touch during examination. Bladder analgesics can be helpful before and after intimacy for both men and women. With intercourse, it is important to communicate with your partner so that they understand your needs and limitations. Often, trying alternative positions is helpful. When you can control the depth of penetration, you can prevent the bladder from getting "bumped" during vaginal intercourse. If the vaginal entrance is tight, gentle massage with a lubricant or dilator can help the muscles relax and allow for more comfortable penetration. It is important to keep an open mind and communicate with your partner to explore other ways of being intimate if vaginal intercourse is not an option.

For those with a muscle/myofascial phenotype or pelvic floor dysfunction, the muscles of the pelvic floor support the bladder and encircle the urethra, vagina, prostate, and rectum. These muscles can cause pain, resulting in urinary symptoms of frequency, urgency, pressure, and spasm. Those with a muscle/myofascial phenotype or pelvic floor dysfunction have muscles that are chronically tense and may have trigger points or painful knots in the muscles or fascia. The vagina will be tight, and it may be painful to have intercourse. With orgasm, the pelvic floor contracts rhythmically. For some, this creates more pain after the climax. Men will often complain of pain in the testicles, perineum, or scrotum during or after ejaculation.

Fortunately, there are several strategies that can ease pain related to the pelvic muscles. Applying heat, stretching the muscles before and after intimacy, and considering the use of muscle relaxers can be beneficial. For women, vaginal dilators are available in assorted sizes in a soft silicone and can relax the opening of the vagina gently and slowly. Using a water-soluble lubricant during dilation is advised. Urinating after dilation is always recommended to help prevent urinary tract infection, even when you have not had sex.

Both men and women may benefit from muscle relaxers such as baclofen, cyclobenzaprine, or vaginal/rectal Valium® to help relax the muscles. Medication can be used either before intimacy or after. Medical marijuana has been helpful both in relaxing the pelvic muscles and managing pain. My patients typically receive the most benefit when they use the combined THC/CBD formulation for intimacy. Overall, these strategies can help individuals manage pain and discomfort associated with pelvic muscle pain during intimacy.

When you have Interstitial Cystitis or Bladder Pain Syndrome, it is common to have difficulty with intimacy. Not only can there be pain or symptom flare-ups related to intimacy, but there can also be sexual dysfunction. Erectile dysfunction, low libido, and difficulty reaching orgasm are all problems that can occur. There are many medications and devices that are used to address erectile dysfunction and low libido. Your healthcare provider should be consulted to determine what options are best for you. Don't be afraid to discuss your concerns, you will be surprised at how many options are available.

Discussing sexual issues with your partner can be challenging, especially in new relationships. However, support groups can provide a safe space for partners to learn more about Interstitial Cystitis and Bladder Pain Syndrome and hear from others with similar experiences.

Living with an unpredictable chronic illness and issues with intimacy can sometimes cause relationship stress. In such cases, seeing a therapist who can address both sexuality and chronic disease can be extremely helpful. A therapist can help you and your partner develop coping strategies to manage the impact of Interstitial Cystitis or Bladder Pain Syndrome on your sex life and overall relationship.

Remember, Interstitial Cystitis or Bladder Pain Syndrome can cause sexual issues that are common and can be managed. Seeking support from healthcare professionals, support groups, and therapists can help you and your partner develop a fulfilling and satisfying sex life despite the challenges of living with a chronic illness.

Chapter 16

Putting It All Together

The concept of phenotyping patients with IC/BPS is a new concept. There is still debate about what the root cause or causes are for IC/BPS. You can ask one clinician, and they may believe that the pelvic floor is the root of all symptoms, and the bladder is just an innocent bystander. Other clinicians feel that this is a problem that has a more central origin, meaning the brain and the nervous system are the causes of the symptoms. They believe that the brain's wiring is responsible for the abnormal perception of the sensations it is receiving. Other clinicians may approach IC/BPS patients as a bladder problem. There are now many papers that are looking at how to phenotype patients. Characteristics such as anesthetic bladder capacity and body mapping of pain are just a couple of examples of ways that patients are being looked at to start separating them into smaller subgroups.

I feel that phenotyping patients into subgroups helps us to look at the smaller groups more closely. It helps us focus on what therapies make sense for each smaller group. We are still developing the idea of phenotyping, and we may identify additional subsets in the future. I have clearly seen that patients I have cared for do fit into these different phenotypes or subsets. This helps explain why different therapies work for one person, but not the next.

The hard part clinically is the overlap between the different phenotypes. Using this subclassification or phenotyping is a starting point that I believe will help shorten the time to develop a plan that works for patients. Why waste time on treatments directed at the bladder when you have a neurological or muscular cause that is outside the bladder? It helps us to think of IC/BPS as not just a bladder problem.

If you have been diagnosed with IC/BPS and have not gotten improvement in your symptoms with therapy, if you have blood in your urine, have a strong history of smoking, if you are 50 years old or older, male, or if you have a history of endometriosis, I feel a cystoscopy is reasonable to do. You need to make sure that endometriosis is not on the bladder. You need to rule out bladder carcinoma if you have a strong smoking history or blood on urinalysis. You need to know if you have ulcers, as there is a therapeutic plan that is specific to this phenotype of patients.

If you have noticed no improvement with therapy, it may be time to reassess the diagnosis. Ulcerative IC is easily diagnosed by cystoscopy. All other patients are diagnosed with BPS by ruling out other causes for the symptoms.

Sometimes we need to reassess the diagnosis.

IC/BPS is an elusive disease or syndrome. We still do not know why it develops, but there continues to be research to help us understand it better. Some of the key points to remember are first that this is a diagnosis of exclusion. Sometimes we label patients with IC/BPS, only to discover years later that there was a different problem that was mimicking IC/BPS.

I had a patient with all the classic symptoms of IC/BPS. Her urine was clear, and examination suggested pain over the bladder; she had hesitancy and occasional flares. She had no food sensitivities. There was no leakage of urine or evidence of nerve or muscle problems. The piece of her history that did not fit perfectly was that she would have more pain with urination and right after urination. She really had no significant relief after she urinated. Slowly, her pain would improve, but she still had an urge to urinate. She felt her stream was getting weaker and weaker. When she did not get relief from typical therapies, I questioned the diagnosis. I brought her to the OR for a cystoscopy and video urodynamics. I performed a cystoscopy and video urodynamics test to fill her bladder with an X-ray contrast and observe her bladder filling and emptying to help determine the cause of her slow stream and elusive symptoms.

As I watched her bladder fill, I could see that she had a pouch or diverticulum under her bladder that was filling with X-ray dye. I found her to have a urethral diverticulum or a pinhole at the beginning of the urethra. A clinician could easily miss this on examination or on a simple cystoscopy. The small opening in her urethra allowed urine to fill a pouch that extended up under her bladder as she would urinate, creating pain in the bladder area and compressing the urethra, which caused her urinary flow to slow (mimicking PFD). As she urinated, the pouch would become more distended, causing more pain. Because this pocket or diverticulum was so high, there was no leakage or post-void drip of urine, which is often seen with a urethral diverticulum. She had the diverticulum removed, and all her symptoms resolved.

The point is, if you are not getting any relief from your symptoms with therapy, it may be time to revisit the diagnosis. When you see a urologist, the tendency is for them to focus on the urinary tract, a gynecologist will focus on the reproductive system, and a physical therapist will focus on the musculature. As clinicians, we need to assess every patient from all angles. So, a multidisciplinary approach can be extremely helpful. A careful history and an open mind are critical.

Roadmaps that summarize potential treatment options for each phenotype.

The roadmaps that I am going to outline are a starting point to help you on your journey to wellness. You should not consider this a medical consultation or medical advice. It is information based on recent research and years of personal experience you can use to see where you fit in based on your symptoms.

Use this as a tool to work with your provider, or to seek additional providers to help develop a multidisciplinary team, if needed. All medications have potential side effects and interactions with other medications. Be aware that even over-the-counter supplements may be contraindicated with certain medical conditions, such as renal insufficiency. Alkalinizing the urine may be contraindicated if you have kidney issues or a history of kidney stones. **Always consult with your provider before changing your treatment plan. Only a clinician that knows your history can counsel you on the ultimate plan to help you on your journey to wellness.**

These roadmaps will hopefully help you explore treatments that your clinician has not yet considered. They may help you get redirected if you have not addressed certain issues. Now is the time to keep an open mind and rethink your diagnosis using this latest information. Information is power, and remember you oversee your journey to wellness.

Chapter 17

Roadmap for Ulcerative Interstitial Cystitis Phenotype

If you have the phenotype of **Ulcerative Interstitial Cystitis**, then you have a disease of the bladder, and we will label you as Interstitial Cystitis. Diet is especially important, as overly acidic urine can feel like vinegar on a canker sore. We recommend going through the process of the elimination diet, as you may be sensitive to certain foods. Alkalinized lidocaine that can be instilled into the bladder with a catheter is helpful for some patients. Patients may be able to instill this at home; others will return to the office for periodic instillations. This approach appears to work well with flare-ups.

The mainstay of therapy in this phenotype is to fulgurate the lesion or Hunner's ulcer with cautery or a laser and/or to inject the steroid triamcinolone into the lesion. Most patients will have a biopsy to confirm that the lesion is not bladder cancer or any other pathology. The biopsy will help guide whether mast cells, eosinophils, or other allergic cells are present. Antihistamines have been immensely helpful in those patients, in my experience. If you still have significant pain or hypersensitivity, then medications that help turn down the nerves can be helpful (amitriptyline, Neurontin®, etc.).

Some providers have used the immunosuppressant cyclosporine A with success in this group. Careful observation for potential adverse reactions is necessary.

Most patients with ulcers will have smaller bladders that just cannot hold much urine, day or night. With treatment of the ulcers, your symptoms may improve enough that you can sometimes stretch the bladder out slowly by doing bladder retraining. This is a method of postponing urination just for a few minutes to improve the bladder capacity gradually. You can find detailed instructions for bladder retraining in the toolbox at the end of the book. Lifestyle changes such as hydration, avoiding constipation, physiological quieting, and proper toileting habits will be beneficial as well.

I have discussed how the body responds to pain and the constant urge to urinate. Many patients with Ulcerative IC will also have pelvic floor dysfunction. Therefore, this should be treated if present. Physical therapy is typically used to treat pelvic floor dysfunction.

Because Ulcerative Interstitial Cystitis occurs more often in older patients, the incidence of genitourinary syndrome of menopause (GSM) is more likely, as are other voiding dysfunctions, such as overactive bladder, prolapse, and incontinence. Men with Ulcerative IC may have underlying prostatic enlargement that may need to be addressed. Medical professionals should evaluate significant prolapse in women, which can create obstruction. If symptoms are present, men should treat prostatic enlargement or clear-cut obstruction from other causes. An evaluation by a urologist will help to determine if there is significant obstruction from prostatic issues.

It is common for patients with ulcers to be more prone to getting urinary tract infections. The ulcers create a rough patch on the bladder wall that allows bacteria to adhere more easily. Hydration is crucial to help prevent overly concentrated urine, which can exacerbate symptoms, as well as to help prevent infections. Using low doses of antibiotics when you are intimate or sexually active has been a successful method of preventing recurrent UTI's in those with documented infections. Consultation with your provider, review of your history, and clear documentation that you have positive urine cultures related to intimacy are all paramount. We usually try therapy with D-mannose, probiotics, treatment for GSM, and hydration first.

Remember that there can be significant overlap in the phenotypes, and it is common to have more than one phenotype. If you identify with any of the other phenotypes, address those issues too. If there are other overlapping syndromes such as vulvodynia, fibromyalgia, or irritable bowel syndrome, then there could be more to the story. You may have a brain-processing phenotype as well. Stress and past trauma or central sensitization syndrome will sidetrack your progress if you ignore the effect your brain has on how you process the signals the bladder is sending.

Some patients in this group will benefit from neuromodulation. The beauty of neuromodulation is that you can evaluate to see if you have benefit or improvement in your symptoms before proceeding with a neurostimulation implant.

To summarize, addressing all the issues and phenotypes present is important to improving symptoms. Fulguration and steroid injections may need to be repeated periodically. You will know when your symptoms require it.

Case presentation:

I initially saw Maureen* at age 62. She had been out to a restaurant for a long dinner with friends. When she went to urinate, the urine was red. I worked her up for visible blood and found that she had a Hunner's ulcer that had bled when the bladder became overdistended. I performed fulguration of the ulcer with a biopsy which showed inflammation and some eosinophils, another type of "allergy" cell in the body. Her history revealed longstanding frequency, but no actual pain. She had been managing her symptoms by limiting fluids if traveling and staying close to a bathroom. I gave her the IC diet, Prelief® as needed, and encouraged her to improve her hydration. She started on an antihistamine and, 10 years later, continues to feel well with only one additional trip to the OR for a fulguration of her ulcer with a steroid injection. She had absolutely no issues with her pelvic floor, and pain was never a significant problem for her. No other phenotypes or associated conditions were present that required treatment. Other similar patients have done well with intermittent treatment of their ulcers, diet, and medications or supplements to help alkalinize the urine should it become too acidic. Bladder retraining can help with frequency once symptoms of pain and urgency are improved with fulguration and/or triamcinolone injection. If the bladder becomes exceedingly small and inelastic, then a handful of patients have gone on to surgery to remove the bladder and create a new urine reservoir, which has significantly helped the intolerable frequency, getting up at night, and pain. This group has the best prognosis with surgery if all else has failed.

Neuromodulation, alternative and complementary therapies if indicated. Consider surgery if small fibrotic bladder and poor quality of life.

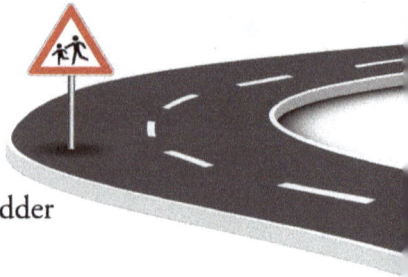

If office cystoscopy done, then proceed to OR: Fulguration and/or triamcinolone recommended. Biopsy if indicated.

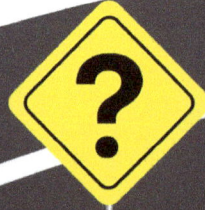

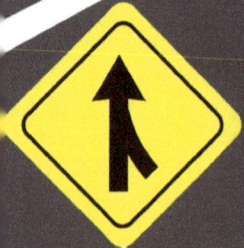

Ulcer has been diagnosed by cystoscopy; Diet important, watch acidic foods. If fulguration and/or triamcinolone done, continue down the road. Physiological quieting, hydration and proper toileting recommended.

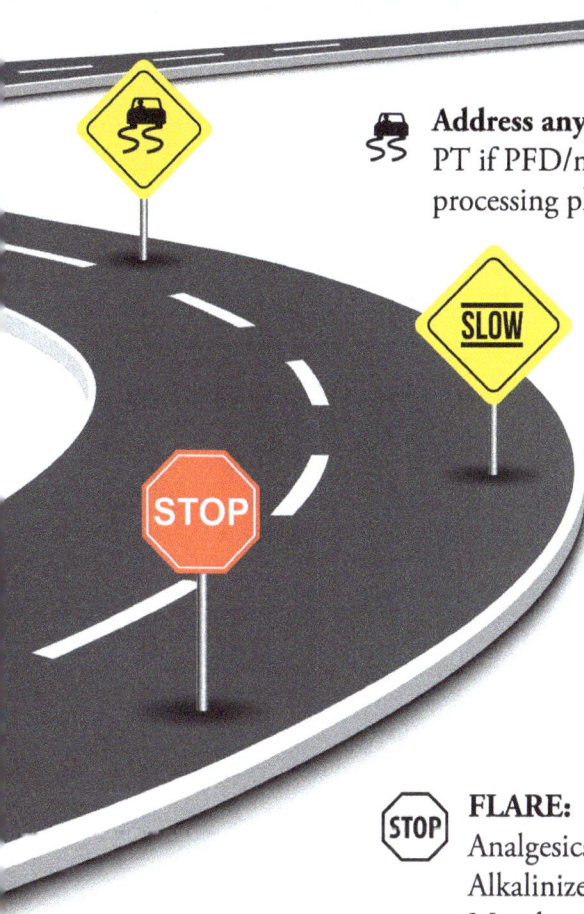

Address any overlapping phenotypes:
PT if PFD/muscle phenotype. Treat brain processing phenotype if present.

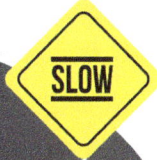

SLOW **Repeat fulguration and/or Triamcinolone as needed.**

STOP **FLARE:**
Analgesics.
Alkalinized lidocaine instillation.
Muscle relaxants if indicated.

? Consider antihistamine if dx shows "allergy cells" and medication if nerve pain (gabapentin, amitriptyline).
Alkalinized lidocaine instillations if needed.
Bladder retraining for frequency.

Roadmap for Ulcerative Interstitial Cystitis

Chapter 18

Roadmap for Bladder Phenotype

If you clearly do not have ulcers, and if you identify your symptoms most closely with a bladder-derived phenotype, then the journey to wellness starts with the simplest treatments first. Diet is important, as the bladder will usually be overly sensitive to foods. Similarly, adequate hydration to prevent concentrated urine is important. Dealing with stress and learning good coping skills and any activity that helps with physiological quieting of the nervous system will be beneficial. Useful techniques include deep breathing, yoga, mindfulness exercises, and meditation. Lifestyle changes that include avoiding constipation, gentle aerobic exercise, and proper toileting habits are all recommended.

If you do a bladder diary, you will usually see a smaller volume with more frequent urination during the day, and at night as well. Because you are urinating to help prevent pain or urgency, the tendency is for the bladder to get smaller and smaller. Once your symptoms improve, bladder retraining is key to reestablishing a better bladder capacity. Typically, we will see pain and urgency improving first, but the improvement in frequency seems to lag. Bladder retraining is a valuable tool that will increase your bladder capacity or the amount of urine that you can hold. This will then help your day and nighttime frequency. The instructions for bladder retraining are available in the toolbox at the end of the book.

A small catheter is used to instill an anesthetic cocktail into the bladder if you are not sure about whether this phenotype fits you. If the bladder is causing your discomfort or pain, you should observe a short-term relief of symptoms while the bladder is numbed.

We still do not know what causes bladder-derived symptoms. Research has shown multiple potential causes. Based on this research, I have narrowed it down to three potential problems. The question is whether it is the GAG layer, the mast cells or histamine and cytokine release, or upregulation of the C-fibers. It is very possible that it is a combination of these factors. For patients that have clear seasonal flares and food sensitivities, you might start with a supplement to help restore the GAG layer and an over-the-counter or prescription antihistamine. If mast cells or histamine excess are issues, then antihistamines, DMSO, amitriptyline, or other medications that stabilize mast cells may be helpful. If pain is a significant component of your symptoms, then medication or instillations that turn the volume down on the nerves and decrease the pain signals can be helpful (amitriptyline, gabapentin and anesthetic cocktails are commonly used).

Patients that have not gotten symptom relief from medications or bladder instillations and have significant frequency will often benefit from medications to relax the bladder or neuromodulation. While neuromodulation is not FDA-approved for the indication of IC/BPS, it has been FDA-approved since 1998 for frequency and urgency. Botox® continues to be explored as a treatment option for this phenotype as well.

We must remember that there is a significant overlap in the phenotypes. Pelvic floor dysfunction is a frequent occurrence which necessitates treatment, usually through physical therapy. We should address any overlapping conditions or symptoms coming from outside of the bladder. Associated conditions, such as GSM, obstruction, overactive bladder, endometriosis, etc., should be addressed.

I have had many patients in this group that have found neuromodulation to be remarkably successful, especially when pelvic floor dysfunction was a significant part of their syndrome or if they had continued frequency and urgency that had not responded to more conservative measures. In many patients, medical marijuana and CBD have been helpful. Vaginal or rectal Valium® has been beneficial, especially post-intimacy, to help prevent flares triggered by sex. Do not be afraid to discuss newer or alternative treatment options with your clinician to create a plan that fits your symptoms and your lifestyle.

It is imperative to regularly evaluate your treatment plan to make sure it is working. Sometimes the improvements are subtle and take time. A bladder diary can show you if things are improving. You should see your bladder is holding a little more, and your frequency is slowly getting better. Clinicians should consider discontinuing treatments that have not been effective. There is some trial and error as you and your clinician try to find the right combination that helps you, so be patient and realize that there may be several factors that need to be addressed before you achieve optimal symptom relief.

I have had many patients achieve almost complete resolution of their symptoms with therapy. Unfortunately, some will go back to their old ways and then trigger a relapse. You may never tolerate diet soda, energy drinks, alcohol, or certain foods. Do not go crazy with your diet once you are in remission. Go slowly and add food and beverages back in moderation. The key here is to consider a multidisciplinary approach to address all coexisting conditions. Gynecological matters must be attended to, musculoskeletal matters must be attended to, and gaining the ability to handle and manage stress is of paramount importance. A healthy lifestyle is important, as well as learning to relax and quiet the nervous system. Try gentle aerobic exercise, stop smoking, and be mindful. Your bladder will thank you.

Case presentation:

Molly* was a young woman who I started treating as a teenager. She had significant frequency, mostly during the day with clear-cut cyclical flares. An evaluation by gynecology revealed no sign of endometriosis. She had microscopic blood in the urine, and the urologic workup, which included a cystoscopy, was negative for any pathology. Medications caused weight gain and drowsiness that was not acceptable as she went through school. She clearly benefited from bladder instillations, which became the mainstay of her therapy, along with diet modifications. She did bladder retraining and increased her bladder capacity. Fast forward, she was married and subsequently had children. She reduced her urinary frequency symptoms, but pain remained an issue, especially with intimacy. Medical marijuana judiciously keeps her symptoms well controlled, and with dietary modifications, relaxation, and support, she continues to do very well. With a flare, she will use a bladder instillation for quick relief. She uses an over-the-counter antihistamine during the spring and fall to help prevent seasonal flare-ups.

Emily* came to me after seeing at least six other doctors. She had tried all typical oral medications and bladder instillations. She was on substantial amounts of narcotics through a pain management doctor but was still suffering and having episodes of retention requiring intermittent catheterization. PT and vaginal Valium® to address her pelvic floor dysfunction had all failed. We tried neuromodulation, and she now urinates normally and has weaned off all narcotics. She still watches her diet and may use antihistamines during seasonal flares but has gotten her life back. She is married and ready to move on.

Consider neuromodulation, Botox®, complementary and alternative therapies. Confirm all overlapping phenotypes and associated conditions have been addressed.

Mast Cell therapy if "allergic" profile. Consider GAG layer therapy, supplement, or PPS. Add medication for C-fiber upregulation if pain significant component, (amitriptyline/gabapentin).

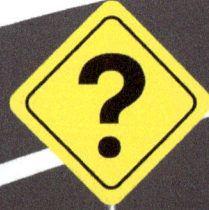

Symptoms are consistent with Bladder derived phenotype; Diet important, watch acidic/trigger foods. Physiological quieting techniques and good bladder and bowel habits are important.

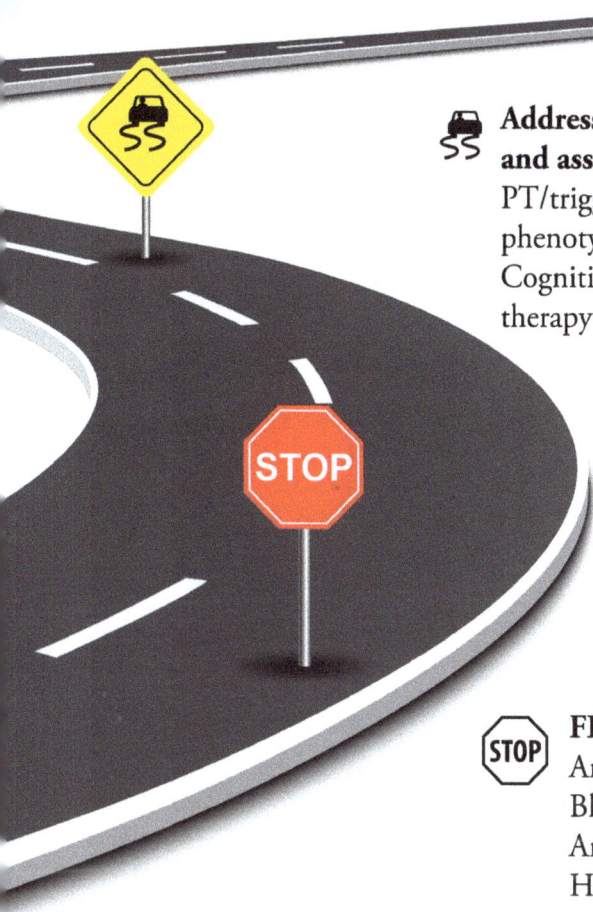

Address any overlapping phenotypes and associated conditions:
PT/trigger point injections for muscle phenotype.
Cognitive behavioral / pain reprocessing therapy for Brain processing phenotype.

FLARE:
Analgesics.
Bladder instillation.
Antispasmodics.
Heat.

? Consider bladder instillation if oral medication not tolerated.
Consider cystoscopy if no improvement to rule out ulcers.
PT if symptoms of PFD.
Bladder Retraining.

Roadmap for Bladder-Derived Phenotype

Chapter 19

Roadmap for Urethral Phenotype

Patients with the urethral phenotype will benefit from following the lifestyle changes previously outlined. Physiological quieting helps to calm overly sensitive nerves, and adequate fiber and hydration helps to avoid constipation. Proper toileting habits will help prevent undo straining with urination, which can exacerbate urethral symptoms. Dietary modifications will be important, as acidic urine will usually exacerbate the urethral pain. Some patients find a low-oxalate diet helpful, as crystals in the urine can exacerbate urethral pain. Similarly, adequate hydration is important to help prevent concentrated urine and crystals in the urine.

We often employ topical treatments for burning at the opening of the urethra. Consider using estrogen cream if peri- or post-menopausal and symptoms of thinning of the tissue are present. Doctors can prescribe topical lidocaine for severe pain or flare-ups. Compounded creams containing combinations of amitriptyline, gabapentin, baclofen, and lidocaine can be helpful. Oral medications used to help turn down the nerve endings, such as amitriptyline or gabapentin, may be beneficial.

Many patients will have pelvic floor dysfunction or a muscle phenotype, and physical therapy may be helpful. Valium® suppositories have been beneficial, sometimes just post-intimacy, or with flares, but some individuals will use them daily to help relax the muscles around the urethra. Other medications that relax the muscles around the urethra are available, and your clinician can counsel you if this is an issue.

Your doctor can administer a nerve block in severe cases. Treatment of other phenotypes is important, as well as evaluation and treatment for other associated conditions. Strictures can present with urethral burning, and slow urinary flow. A urethral diverticulum can mimic IC/BPS, so cystoscopy or additional testing may be indicated if no improvement occurs with initial therapy. Your doctor may consider giving a trial of antibiotics if there is concern about possible urethritis.

Case presentation:

Betsy* was a 70-year-old woman with frequent severe episodes of urethral pain, often associated with a feeling of incomplete emptying. She felt like she had vaginitis or a urinary tract infection. The symptoms would come on suddenly and often would prompt a visit to the ER to gain relief. Her urine cultures were routinely negative, and usually, vaginal swabs would come back normal. She struggled with constipation and, when severe, had hesitancy to urinate. Review of a bladder diary showed limited fluid intake and smaller-than-normal bladder volumes during the day. No other findings were present on examination other than thinning of the vaginal tissue, consistent with menopause, and tenderness over the urethra and pelvic floor. An X-ray was performed to rule out a urethral diverticulum and was normal. Cystoscopy was normal, with no Hunner's ulcers or lesions present.

Betsy was started on the IC elimination diet, and hydration was improved. Urinalysis was consistently acidic, so Prelief® was added. She was started on a topical estrogen cream to treat the vaginal and urethral tissue thinning. She addressed her constipation and was taught to relax her pelvic muscles with urination and bowel movements. A Squatty Potty® was used to help with pelvic floor relaxation. Finally, the use of a compounded cream with baclofen, amitriptyline, lidocaine, and gabapentin applied at the opening of the vagina and urethra helped to turn down the nerve endings, and she found relief. Now with a flare, she alkalinizes the urine, increases hydration, and will apply a lidocaine ointment to the meatus. The frequency of severe flares has decreased, and she is now working on bladder retraining to improve her bladder capacity. She continues to improve.

Consider nerve block if symptoms persist. Confirm other potential pathology such as strictures or urethral diverticulum ruled out.

Topical cream to meatus and vaginal opening. Topical lidocaine. Compounded cream to turn down nerve endings (gabapentin, amitriptyline, baclofen may be used).

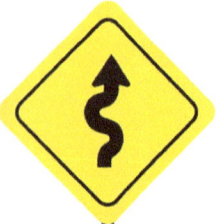

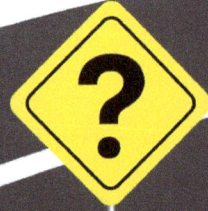

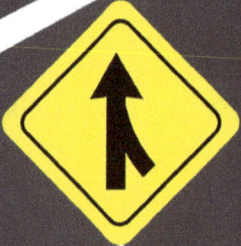

Symptoms are consistent with Urethral phenotype; Diet important, watch acidic/trigger foods.
Hydration very important. Physiological quieting techniques and good bladder and bowel habits are important.

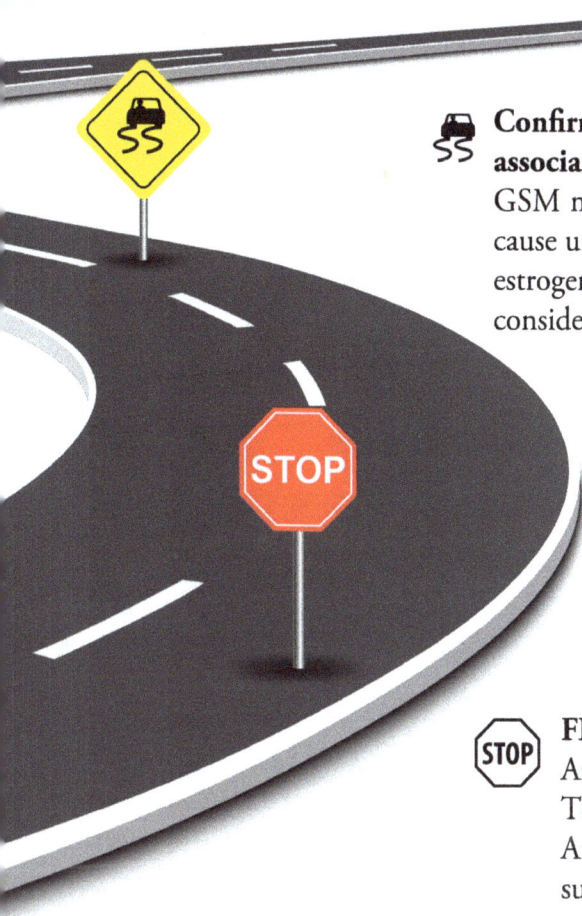

Confirm overlapping phenotypes and associated conditions are treated.
GSM must be addressed as this can also cause urethral symptoms, topical estrogen or alternative should be considered.

FLARE:
Analgesics.
Topical lidocaine.
Antispasmodics such as Valium® suppository.

Consider cystoscopy if no improvement to rule out other pathology.
PT if symptoms of PFD.
Consider oral muscle relaxants if spasm.
Consider medications to turn down nerves if pain persists (gabapentin, amitryptiline).
Bladder Retraining if frequency persists.

Roadmap for Urethral Phenotype

Chapter 20

Roadmap for Infection Phenotype

Patients with the infection phenotype follow a similar roadmap to the bladder phenotype. Everyone should follow the lifestyle changes outlined previously. Physiological quieting is emphasized as C-fiber hypersensitivity has been shown to occur with chronic infections. Dietary modification is recommended, as there is usually bladder inflammation and nerve upregulation present. Adequate hydration is important, as concentrated urine will worsen symptoms. Adequate hydration is also very important to help prevent future infections.

Treatment is based primarily on symptoms and clues to potential contributing factors. Doctors may prescribe antihistamines if they suspect mast cell overactivity. If there is evidence of C-fiber upregulation and pain, then medications to turn down the nerves such as amitriptyline or gabapentin may be helpful. Bladder instillations can be used but can trigger infections in some patients. You may consider supplements to support the GAG layer.

Measures to help prevent recurrent urinary tract infections, such as D-mannose, hydration, probiotics, and treatment for genitourinary syndrome of menopause, should be considered. Prophylactic antibiotics may help if documented infections occur during intimacy or other activities.

Clinicians should address all overlapping phenotypes. It is common to see pelvic floor dysfunction, in which case physical therapy would be helpful.

If frequency, urgency, and pain persist, and more conservative therapies have failed, cystoscopy should be considered if it has never been done, to rule out a Hunner's ulcer or lesion, as well as other causes for recurrent infections. If symptoms persist, and conservative therapies have failed, then neuromodulation and alternative therapies are an option.

Case presentation:

Sally* was a young woman that was sent to me with recurrent urinary tract infections. These were not always cultured and were often treated on the weekends with an empiric trial of antibiotics. Review of her history showed poor fluid intake and frequent urination during the day, less so at night. She described a dull pressure in the bladder region that improved after she urinated. Often, her UTI symptoms occurred the week before her period. She also had severe cramping and pain with her periods. She had pain with intercourse. She also had vaginal discharge and had been treated for bacterial vaginitis as well as yeast infections.

Sally was referred to her gynecologist for evaluation and to rule out endometriosis that might be mimicking the UTI symptoms on a cyclical basis. She was given a trial of oral contraceptives to see if the gynecologic symptoms would improve, and they did somewhat. She was started on a probiotic to help improve the vaginal flora and was given a list of dietary irritants to avoid. Her hydration improved. She was given lab slips and a urine culture cup so that she could always get a urine culture (UC) if symptoms arose. She was given a prophylactic antibiotic to use post-intercourse. Our goal was to keep her infection-free for three months, and to improve the good bacteria that surrounded the urethra. Slowly, her symptoms improved, but she still had mild bladder discomfort that caused frequency. Low-dose amitriptyline was added at bedtime, to help turn down overly sensitive nerves. Symptoms improved, and after six months, she was able to wean off the amitriptyline. Now she is symptom-free, but continues with good hydration, dietary modifications, and a probiotic.

If infections have been controlled and symptoms persist, despite conservative therapy, consider neuromodulation, complementary and alternative treatments.

Mast Cell therapy if "allergic" profile.
Consider GAG layer therapy with supplement.
Add medication for C-fiber upregulation if pain significant component (amitriptyline/gabapentin).
Regimen to prevent future infections, based on history.

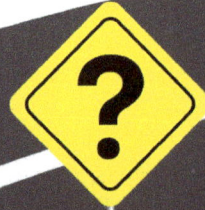

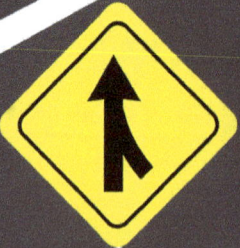

Symptoms are consistent with Infection phenotype; Diet and hydration are important, watch acidic/trigger foods. Physiological quieting techniques and good bladder and bowel habits are important. Must do Urine culture to confirm infections.

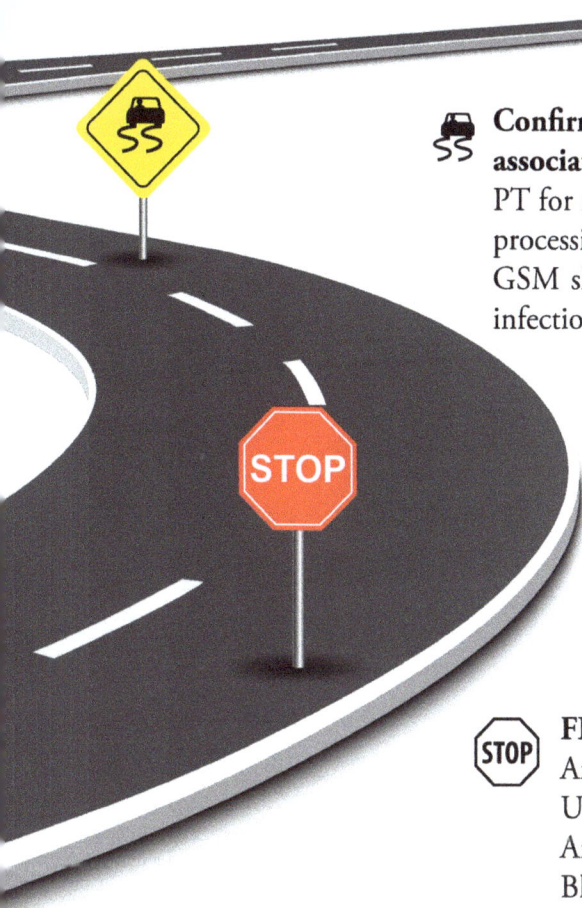

Confirm overlapping phenotypes and associated conditions are treated.
PT for muscle phenotype. Brain processing phenotype addressed. GSM should be treated to help prevent infections.

FLARE:
Analgesics.
UC and antibiotics if indicated.
Antispasmodics.
Bladder instillation if has had favorable response in past.

Consider bladder instillation if oral medications not tolerated.
Consider cystoscopy if no improvement to rule out ulcers or other pathology.
PT if symptoms of PFD.
Bladder Retraining.
UC if symptoms of UTI.

Roadmap for Infection Phenotype

Chapter 21

Roadmap for Muscle or Myofascial phenotype

You fit into this phenotype if you have primarily a muscle or myofascial problem. You may have a history of trauma, either physical or emotional. Patients may notice that they have frequency during the day but can hold a more normal volume in their bladder at night. Foods rarely trigger symptoms as much. If you have had a bladder instillation with lidocaine, you may notice that it really did not change your discomfort or pain. It is common to have constipation or difficulty evacuating your bowels even when they are soft. Sometimes you may have hesitancy or must sit and relax to get your stream started. You may have tenderness in the muscles on examination, or trigger points that are tender and may reproduce the urinary symptoms when touched. If this is your primary problem, then the symptoms are coming from outside the bladder, and the muscles or fascia are the primary problem.

As with all phenotypes, there may be overlap, and any other phenotypes will need to be addressed. If there has been a history of abuse, or if you have other chronic overlapping conditions such as fibromyalgia, vulvodynia, irritable bowel, prostadynia, or central sensitization syndrome, your brain may not be processing the signals that it receives properly. This, as well as other psychological conditions such as PTSD, depression, or anxiety, may need to be addressed to get optimal relief from your symptoms.

The starting point for patients with a muscle/myofascial phenotype is physical therapy and lifestyle changes. It is important to avoid constipation. Every individual should take heed of the lifestyle changes recommended previously. Physiological quieting techniques and proper toileting habits are especially important. Many patients find the Squatty Potty® helpful to relax the pelvic muscles when urinating or moving the bowels.

Learning to quiet the nervous system will help to quiet the muscles. Learning to deal with stress and develop good coping skills will help to quiet the muscles. Stretching, yoga, tai chi, and Reiki therapy all can help calm an overly stressed system.

If there are specific tender spots or trigger points, then trigger point injections can be helpful. Some individuals do well with Botox® injections into the pelvic floor or other affected areas to help relax specific muscles. Many patients find that muscle relaxants, such as baclofen or Valium® suppositories, either vaginally or rectally, are beneficial. Clinicians may prescribe Valium® suppositories daily or just with a flare-up.

Neuromodulation has worked well in this group of patients, especially if retention has been an issue. Because this is a more invasive procedure, we do it after we have tried all less invasive treatments. Alternative therapies such as acupuncture, TENS units, and medical marijuana have been helpful for some patients.

With a muscle/myofascial phenotype, a multidisciplinary team is crucial. Because physical therapy is a key component to treating this subset, finding a therapist that has expertise in treating the pelvic floor is important. Biofeedback can be a useful tool to help with conscious relaxation of the pelvic muscles, especially when you are urinating or moving the bowels. We recommend avoiding Kegel or strengthening exercises, as this can make your symptoms worse.

Case presentation:

Sally* is a 20-year-old woman that had a traumatic sexual experience. Her gynecologist noticed no obvious physical trauma, but Sally started having problems with both her urination and her bowels. She had difficulty relaxing to move her bowels and started having constant pelvic pain and urinary frequency. She had frequent, small-volume urination during the day but would often sleep through the night without having to urinate. She did not notice any change in her symptoms with diet. She grew increasingly frustrated as she was told over and over that her urine was clear and that there was nothing wrong. Her gynecologist sent her to me for an evaluation of the urinary symptoms. On examination, it was apparent that she had significant muscle tightness and tenderness of the pelvic floor muscles. A combination of psychological support and physical therapy improved her symptoms significantly. She is now doing bladder retraining, and the frequency has improved. She is continuing with psychological counseling because of the trauma she experienced, which has been extremely helpful in getting her back on her path to wellness.

I was referred Claire* at age 38 after multiple hernia operations and pelvic surgeries. She had significant straining to urinate or move her bowels. She continued to have severe pelvic pain. Foods did not aggravate her symptoms. She had a complicated medical history because of spinal issues and multiple back and pelvic operations. She had a decreased bladder capacity on a bladder diary, and cystoscopy showed no ulcers. Urodynamics showed that her pelvic muscles did not relax when she urinated. Typical treatments directed at bladder-derived Bladder Pain Syndrome did not benefit her. A combination of muscle relaxants, vaginal Valium®, physical therapy, and psychological support to address her chronic overlapping conditions has improved her symptoms. Chronic pain in her spine and pelvis continues to be a problem, and pain management has been helpful for her. She is now 64, and it is her back pain that limits her the most.

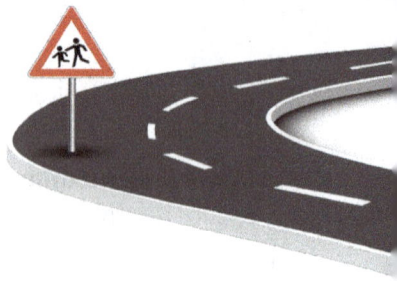

Physical Therapy, trigger point injections if needed. Consider muscle relaxants.

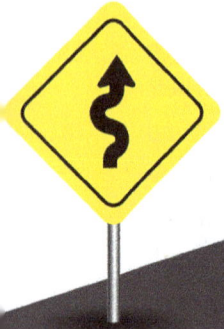

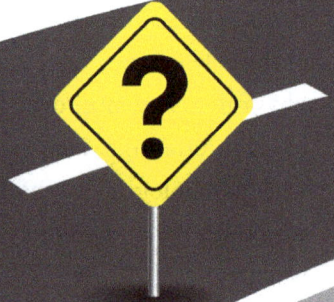

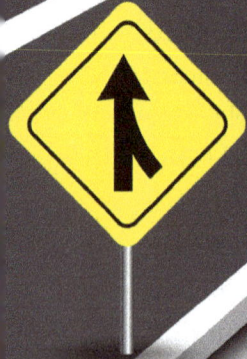

Physical Exam or symptoms consistent with primary muscle/myofascial phenotype. Physiological quieting techniques and proper bowel and bladder habits, avoid constipation.

Consider Neuromodulation.
Complementary or alternative treatments.

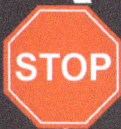

FLARE:
Heat.
Muscle Relaxers.
Analgesics.
Lidocaine patch.

Address overlapping phenotypes or associated conditions.
Consider Botox®/ additional trigger point injections.

Roadmap for Muscle or Myofascial Phenotype

Chapter 22

Roadmap for the Neuralgia Phenotype

This group of patients is the least common that I have seen in my practice as a primary phenotype. When I have seen it, it is usually obvious. Patients will present with significant pain that is sharper and usually more focused. Sometimes it is more severe on one side. Patients typically describe the pain as sharp, occasionally shooting into the leg, often feeling like a vibration or electrical sensation. Patients have come into my office for consultation and asked to stay standing as we talk. Some have come in with a pillow to sit on. Sometimes, there is a clear history of long bike rides or trauma that is linked to the onset of symptoms. The frequency and urgency seem to develop after the pain, whereas in bladder-derived phenotypes, the frequency and urgency seem to start first, with pain developing later. Bladder diaries have been variable. Some will have only a mild decrease in bladder volumes in a diary, and foods rarely cause an increase in symptoms. I often see signs of muscle tightness in this group, such as urinary hesitancy or slow flow, which may be a secondary pelvic floor dysfunction. Other patients have a history of a muscle/myofascial phenotype first and seem to develop neuralgia symptoms later. Examination typically will show significant tenderness over the pudendal nerve and at times the pelvic muscles.

If clinicians suspect pudendal neuralgia or a neurologic cause, then they must consider further testing to rule out a structural cause for the pain. An MRI can be useful in this scenario. I have used neurology and pain management for a pudendal nerve block to help with both diagnosis and treatment. We recommend physical therapy and lifestyle changes initially. Avoiding activities that irritate the pudendal nerve, such as horseback riding, squatting, and protracted sitting or cycling, are helpful. Some have experienced an improvement in their symptoms when using TENS units. Medications that stabilize the nerves or antiseizure medications like gabapentin may help with nerve pain. A lidocaine patch can be helpful with a flare. Some have used Botox® injections into the muscles affected. Pudendal neuromodulation has shown excellent results for patients with pudendal neuralgia.[59] Sometimes, surgery to decompress the nerve is recommended. However, it is only done in a few select centers, with relief after surgery sometimes taking years.

Case presentation:

Helen* was a 48-year-old female that came in with persistent urinary frequency and pain in the perineum (area between the lower buttocks and vagina) and lower bladder area. She felt shooting pains and a feeling of swelling in the vagina. She was having more frequency and pressure to urinate. The symptoms had been ongoing for several months. She had altered her lifestyle drastically, taking up long-distance biking on the weekends and cycling to and from work about 20 miles each day. Symptoms of pain increased as the day went on, with more pain in the evenings. Her pain was worse if sitting at her desk, so she started standing to work. She experienced considerable pain when the pudendal nerve on the right side was palpated, and no other vaginal

---

59   Peters KM, et al: Chronic pudendal neuromodulation: expanding available treatment options for refractory urologic symptoms. NeuroUrol. Urody 2010; 29(7): 1267-71.

swelling or anomalies were observed on examination. Her bladder diary showed only slightly decreased bladder capacity. She stopped bicycling completely. The pain management doctor performed a pudendal nerve block that provided her with significant relief, and she repeated it several times. She was prescribed gabapentin and started physical therapy. Her urinary symptoms improved, and the pain resolved. The following spring, she tried bicycling again, this time in moderation and with a new bike seat with a central cut-out, designed to prevent pressure on the perineum. She continues to do well.

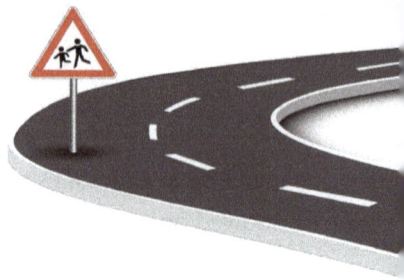

Physical Therapy.
Pudendal nerve block both for diagnosis and therapy of pudendal neuralgia.
Medications to quiet nerve pain.
Analgesics.

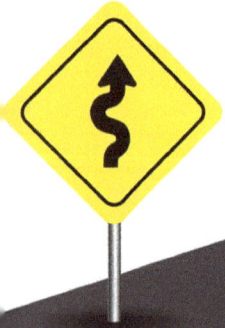

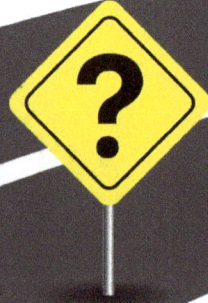

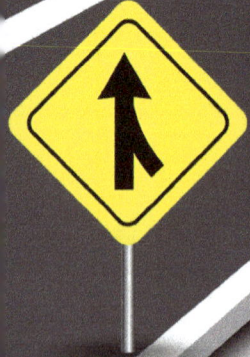

Symptoms are consistent with Neuralgia phenotype; Physiological quieting techniques and good bladder and bowel habits are important.
Eliminate or modify activities that may be contributing to symptoms.
Additional diagnostic testing to rule out other pathology if indicated.

Consider neuromodulation, alternative and complementary therapies, i.e., TENS unit, acupuncture, medical marijuana. Surgery for nerve entrapment available in select centers.

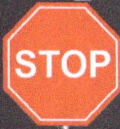

FLARE:
Analgesics.
Lidocaine patch.
Antispasmodics.
Heat.
Medications to decrease nerve pain.

Address overlapping phenotypes and associated conditions:
Repeat pudendal nerve block if benefited from initial block.
Continue with PT/trigger point injections if needed.

Roadmap for Neuralgia Phenotype

Chapter 23

Roadmap for Brain-Processing Phenotype

Multiple Pain Disorders/Central Sensitization Syndrome

This is the most complex group of patients to treat. The connection between the brain and the signals that it receives is incredibly complicated. Fortunately, this is an area of increased interest and research, so hopefully, more answers will be forthcoming soon. Multiple complaints and symptoms characterize this phenotype, often outside of the bladder and pelvic area. There may be multiple chronic overlapping pain conditions, such as irritable bowel syndrome, migraines, fibromyalgia, temporomandibular pain, vulvodynia, chronic fatigue syndrome, and prostadynia, to name a few. Patients usually describe the bladder or pelvic pain as severe, like a knife or hot poker. Often, this is associated with significant anxiety or depression. There may be signs of hypersensitivity to foods, chemicals, smells, sounds, or environmental allergens. Patients may be prone to rashes and hot or cold sensitivity. Usually, they have seen many doctors, and some have had many surgeries trying to find relief.

There is good evidence that the brain has changed and become more hypersensitive in these individuals. These individuals experience an intensification of pain perception and may also display anxiety, catastrophizing, and depression. I am not saying that this is a mental illness; it is a brain that, when stimulated, is overreacting negatively. Fortunately, there are ways to rewire how the brain responds to the signals that it receives.

The key here is to embrace a multidisciplinary approach. Clearly, lifestyle changes are important. Activities that quiet the nervous system like meditation, deep breathing, mindfulness techniques, gentle aerobic exercise, and yoga are all helpful. Dietary modification to eliminate bladder irritants is important, as is adequate hydration. Physical therapy should be used to address pelvic floor dysfunction or muscle/myofascial phenotype. Medications that help to relieve muscle spasms can be used. Some patients will tolerate anesthetic bladder cocktails and find some relief. If marked environmental hypersensitivity is noted, antihistamines could be helpful.

Cognitive-behavioral and pain reprocessing therapies can help to change how the brain perceives the signals that it receives and is an important part of therapy. Fortunately, our brains are capable of neuroplasticity and can be retrained to respond differently. A program that helps to calm the nervous system will help to restore good brain function and decrease the hypersensitive response that can affect multiple systems in the body. In addition, doctors may use medications to help turn down upregulated nerves. Invasive procedures may have a negative impact on therapy by creating more pain and symptoms. Treatment of central brain-processing upregulation and any underlying depression, anxiety, or PTSD is especially important.

It may be hard to tell what other phenotypes exist in the initial presentation. Therefore, starting the journey to wellness starts with the brain and its responses to the stimuli it receives. After this step, it will become easier to determine if there are other phenotypes present. If there are other chronic overlapping pain conditions, improvement may be seen with the therapies listed above. A multidisciplinary approach is important, as many organ systems are involved.

Case presentation:

I initially saw Brianna* as a young woman. She had seen many other doctors and had tried many treatments focused on the bladder. She experienced severe frequency, pelvic pain, migraines, irritable bowel disease, and vulvodynia. She had severe pain during intercourse, which had caused several failed relationships. She had significant anxiety about her future. She had symptoms of pelvic floor dysfunction with intermittent hesitancy and had been to the ER with retention many times. She was seeing a pain management doctor and was on high doses of narcotics and antianxiety medications. We tried physical therapy, but she thought it was too painful, so she stopped going. She was initially very resistant to referral for evaluation by a psychologist, but finally agreed. She gained coping mechanisms over time, took up relaxation tactics, and tackled stress and anxiety. We adjusted her medications, and her pain improved. She tried PT again and was successful. She started a new relationship with an incredibly supportive partner and was married. Her outlook on life improved, and she wanted to become pregnant. This required total refocusing for her, but she came off all narcotics and her other medications that were contraindicated during her pregnancy and used the support of her therapist to work even harder on quieting her nervous system. She now has two children and is on no medications other than occasional medical marijuana and vaginal Valium® after intercourse.

The key to her successful outcome was finally being open to understanding that her brain's response to stimuli was abnormal and overly sensitive. She was able, through hard work and perseverance, to quiet her nervous system and learn to cope better. Unfortunately, many patients will not take this step and do not understand it is not always a bladder problem or a bowel problem, etc. A brain that is hypersensitive will affect multiple areas of the body, but you can change it. As I mentioned at the beginning, there is growing research on the brain's role in chronic overlapping pain conditions, of which IC/BPS is one. There is hope that we will learn more about how to better treat this challenging group of individuals.

Neuromodulation, complementary and alternative therapies.

Confirm all phenotypes addressed as well as other conditions such as OAB, GSM, obstruction.

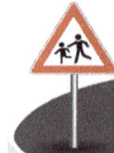

Mast Cell therapy if "allergic" profile or central sensitization syndrome.

Add medication for C-fiber upregulation if pain significant component.

Consider referral to psychologist for cognitive behavioral/pain reprocessing therapy and assessment.

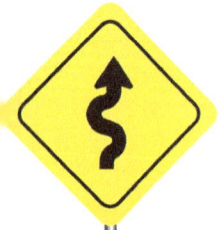

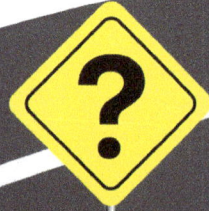

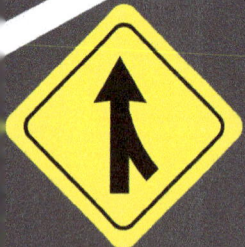

Symptoms are consistent with Brain processing phenotype;
Diet important. Physiological quieting techniques and good bladder and bowel habits are important.

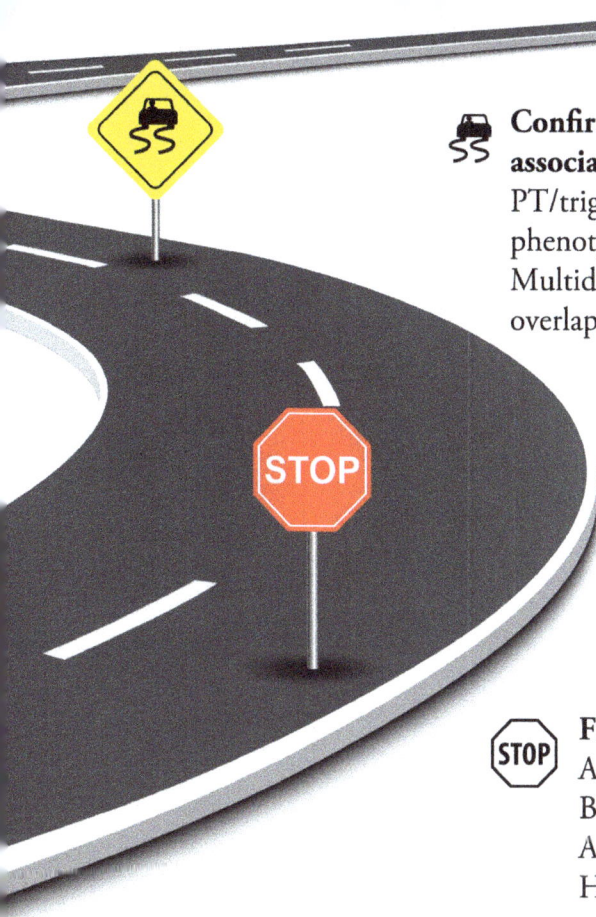

Confirm overlapping phenotypes and associated conditions are treated.

PT/trigger point injections for muscle phenotype.

Multidisciplinary approach to chronic overlapping pain syndromes.

FLARE:
Analgesics.
Bladder instillation.
Antispasmodics.
Heat.

PT if symptoms of PFD/muscle phenotype.
Anesthetic bladder instillation if tolerated and severe bladder pain.

Roadmap for Brain-Processing Phenotype

Part IV

Treatments in Detail, Final Thoughts, and Toolbox

This section will delve into the various treatments that we have discussed, providing more detailed information. We will also explore alternative therapies and nontraditional options. Hopefully, this information will be helpful to you and your healthcare provider, as you consider treatment options that you may not have considered in the past. I will also provide you with some final thoughts about IC/BPS and the exciting research that is ongoing. Finally, the toolbox provides you with questionnaires to monitor treatment progress, the bladder diary, and instructions for bladder retraining. There are other tools that you may find useful as well. If you require further information on specific topics, I have provided a resource guide for your convenience.

Chapter 24

Treatments in Detail

Lifestyle changes

We have covered how several lifestyle changes can be beneficial for patients with IC/BPS. These include maintaining a healthy diet, regular gentle aerobic exercise, stretching, practicing physiological quieting techniques, establishing good bathroom habits, applying heat or cold to painful areas, and staying well hydrated. Taking part in support groups can provide both emotional support and a safe place to discuss concerns. Seek out local support groups as well as online support groups. It is important to manage stress and develop skills to help you cope and better deal with the challenges of a chronic illness. The goal is to achieve remission so there are minimal symptoms, and these lifestyle changes will help to achieve and maintain those improvements.

Physical therapy

Clinicians and researchers believe that up to 87 percent of patients with IC/BPS have the muscle or myofascial phenotype, which includes pelvic floor dysfunction, either as a primary phenotype or secondary. Pelvic floor dysfunction is common as the muscles tense in response to the constant urge to urinate or in response to pain. It is also possible that pelvic floor dysfunction causes the urgency and pain. Either way, the focus is on treatment with physical therapy.

Physical therapy by clinicians trained to treat IC/BPS, and specifically myofascial pain syndrome and pelvic floor dysfunction, is paramount. Physical therapists should be specially trained to perform internal myofascial release if indicated.

Physical therapy is tailored to each patient based on an individual evaluation by the physical therapist, including assessing for any history of trauma. Treatment may include targeted internal (pelvic) and external trigger point treatments. Physical therapy focuses on the muscles and connective tissues of the pelvic floor, as well as the hip girdle and abdomen. Therapy may include connective tissue manipulation of the abdominal wall, hips, and thighs. The therapist stretches the muscles and educates patients on how to relax the pelvic floor and other affected muscles. Treating the tenderness and tightness of the pelvic floor or other muscles can positively affect the bladder, bowel, and genitourinary symptoms. Physical therapists can treat trigger points, scarring, and muscle spasm with a variety of treatments, individualized based on their assessment of each unique patient.

It is important to note that pelvic floor strengthening exercises, such as Kegel exercises, should be avoided, as they can exacerbate symptoms.

Oral medications

Pentosan polysulfate sodium (PPS) or Elmiron® is an FDA-approved medication felt to help restore the bladder's glycosaminoglycan (GAG) layer. Studies have shown that a subset of patients have experienced relief from their IC/BPS symptoms after taking Elmiron®.

However, it is important to note that Elmiron® can have side effects, including diarrhea, hair loss, nausea, headache, stomach upset, and abdominal pain. Elmiron® acts as a mild blood thinner, which can lead to easy bruising or bleeding. Because of the blood thinning properties, patients may need to discontinue use of Elmiron® prior to certain surgeries.

Recent studies have revealed concerns about the prolonged use of Elmiron® and the development of pigmentary maculopathy in patients. Patients should consider the risks and benefits when starting and continuing Elmiron®. I have counseled patients that have benefited from Elmiron® to use the lowest effective dose possible or to consider changing to a supplement that may help to restore the GAG layer.

According to the provisions specified in Chapter 7, if individuals choose to remain on Elmiron®, they should receive ophthalmologic evaluation and follow-up. If a patient has had a favorable response to Elmiron®, they may consider switching to an off-label intravesical instillation of the medication or try a supplement that may improve the GAG layer. Intravesical hyaluronic acid is available in Canada and Europe.

Cimetidine is a compound created in 1971, which blocks histamine H2 receptors. Remember that the mast cells release histamine in response to various triggers. Cimetidine suppresses the production of gastric acid and is most often used to alleviate heartburn and treat peptic ulcers. Its use in IC/BPS facilitates the stabilization of mast cells in patients possessing bladder phenotypes where mast cell activation is believed to be a challenge. Cimetidine can interact with certain medications due to its effects on enzymes in the body that metabolize or break down other medications. Cimetidine must be taken with caution when combined with tricyclic antidepressants like amitriptyline and with gabapentin. It may decrease the effects of codeine, tramadol, and tamoxifen. There are some small studies using cimetidine in IC/BPS patients, but given the potential to interact with other drugs, this medication is listed as an option under the AUA guidelines.[60] I have

60   Clemens JC, Erickson DR, Varela NP, and Lai HH: Diagnosis and treatment of interstitial cystitis/bladder pain syndrome; J. Urol 2022; 208: 34-42.

not found cimetidine to be helpful and choose other antihistamine drugs with fewer drug interactions.

Hydroxyzine is a prescription antihistamine. Hydroxyzine HCl (Atarax®) and hydroxyzine pamoate (Vistaril®) are both commonly used to treat patients with IC/BPS. We typically use it in adults and children to relieve itching from allergic skin conditions. It can also relieve anxiety and tension. It often causes drowsiness, which may help IC/BPS patients with nighttime frequency. Because it can make you drowsy, I use it only at night and in small doses. This medication is prescribed for Ulcerative Interstitial Cystitis and bladder-derived phenotype patients exhibiting signs of mast cell hyperactivity or histamine abundance. It may also be used in patients with central sensitization syndrome with multiple allergies.

Amitriptyline is a tricyclic antidepressant. It works by raising the levels of important chemicals in the brain that affect your mood, like serotonin and norepinephrine. Developed initially as an antidepressant, it is now seldom used for that purpose, as there are newer, more effective antidepressants available. We use amitriptyline outside its labeling to treat nerve pain and ward off migraines. The usual side effects are sluggishness, constipation, and a greater appetite, potentially leading to weight gain. It is prescribed in patients with Ulcerative Interstitial Cystitis and bladder-derived phenotype patients who are suspected to have mast cells overstimulated or hypersensitive C-fibers.

Clinicians also prescribe amitriptyline to manage pain, so it can be useful in myofascial/muscle and neuralgia phenotypes as well. Some patients with the brain phenotype will do well with amitriptyline. It has a mild antihistamine effect that helps those with mast cell issues. Amitriptyline also has mild bladder-relaxing properties. AUA guidelines list amitriptyline as an option for treatment of IC/BPS. Patients should take it at night in the lowest dose that is effective to minimize the risk of side effects.

Cromolyn sodium (Gastrocrom® and Nasalcrom®) is a mast cell stabilizer. It helps to prevent the release of histamine and cytokines or cell-to-cell communicators. It is FDA-approved for the prophylaxis of mild to moderate bronchial asthma. It is also used to help treat allergic rhinitis and systemic mast cell disease (mastocytosis). It has been used off-label in the management of inflammatory bowel disease.

Gabapentin/pregabalin are anticonvulsant medications. Gabapentin or Neurontin® is typically used to treat partial seizures and neuropathic pain. It is a first-line therapy in the treatment of neuropathic pain caused by diabetic neuropathy, postherpetic neuralgia seen with shingles, and central pain. There is evidence that a combination of gabapentin and an opioid or nortriptyline may work better than either drug alone.[61] Dizziness and drowsiness are the most common side effects. It may cause weight gain for some patients. It has been reported to cause difficulty with orgasm or erectile dysfunction which reverses after stopping the medication.

Pregabalin or Lyrica® is a drug that has anticonvulsant, analgesic, and antianxiety properties, which is prescribed to treat epilepsy, neuropathic pain, fibromyalgia, restless leg syndrome, opioid withdrawal, and generalized anxiety disorder. Common side effects include headache, dizziness, sleepiness, dry mouth, blurred vision, and weight gain. Erectile dysfunction may occur as well. An increased risk of suicide may occur, and addiction can happen if taken in high doses. In the US it is a Schedule V controlled substance.

Cyclosporine A is an immunosuppressant. Clinicians often prescribe it to counteract rejection following certain transplants. We also use it in rheumatoid arthritis and psoriasis. Clinicians have used it for chronic hives, systemic mastocytosis, and ulcerative colitis. This medication is rarely prescribed but is listed as an alternative specifically for patients with Ulcerative Interstitial Cystitis who show no improvement from

---

61   Attal N, Cruccu G, Baron R, Haanppaa M, et al: EFNS guideline on the pharmacological treatment of neuropathic pain: 2010 revision; Euro. J. of Neurology 2010; 17(9): 1113-e88.

fulguration and/or triamcinolone injection. This medication requires close monitoring due to potentially serious side effects. Side effects include high blood pressure, elevated potassium, kidney, and liver dysfunction. There is an increased vulnerability to infections. There is an increased risk of squamous cell skin cancer and non-Hodgkin lymphoma. Many urologists will refer patients to other providers that use cyclosporine A more often and have experience in following patients on this medication.

Over-the-counter antihistamines such as Zyrtec®, Claritin®, Allegra® and Benadryl® will also help some patients with allergic symptoms and evidence of mast cell excess, or histamine excess. Most patients will tolerate non-drowsy options.

Nutraceuticals such as calcium glycerophosphate or Prelief®, and supplements containing Aloe Vera, quercetin, and hyaluronic acid, are available. These supplements have some data suggesting improvement in symptoms. Prelief® works as a urinary buffer to neutralize acid in the urine.

The supplements that contain quercetin and hyaluronic acid may help with GAG layer integrity. Examples of these supplements are Cysta Q®, CystoRenew®, or CystoProtek® to name a few. Desert Harvest Aloe vera may also help to restore the GAG layer and improve symptoms. Well-controlled, large studies on these drugs is limited. Patients with bladder-derived phenotypes with GAG layer deficiency as a potential contributing factor may benefit from these supplements.

Palmitoylethanolamide (PEA), PEAORA®, Bladder Builder®, or AloePath® is a supplement that is derived from fat. It is an endocannabinoid-like lipid mediator with extensively documented anti-inflammatory, analgesic, antimicrobial, immunomodulatory, and neuroprotective effects.[62] It has been found to be helpful in treating IC/BPS patients that have not responded to other therapies. Approximately

---

62   Clayton P, Hill M, Bogoda N, Subah S, Venkatesh R. Palmitoylethanolamide: A natural compound for health management. Int. J. Mol. Sci. 2021 May 18; 22(10): 5305.

86 percent of patients noted significant reduction in pain after using it for three months. Combining PEA with aloe or other ingredients seems to work as well if not better. Well-controlled, large studies are limited and data on long-term usage is sparse.

Analgesics, non-narcotic: The most used non-narcotic analgesics in the US are acetaminophen or Tylenol®, ibuprofen or Motrin®, and aspirin. It is important to follow the recommended dosage on the label and consult with your provider if you have liver or kidney issues or are on a blood thinner. Naproxen or Aleve® is another non-narcotic analgesic with a longer effect than ibuprofen, acetaminophen, or aspirin.

Narcotic analgesics include hydrocodone, oxycodone, morphine, fentanyl, codeine, hydromorphone (Dilaudid®) and meperidine (Demerol®). Methadone and buprenorphine are additional narcotic drugs. Narcotic analgesics work by activating opioid receptors, producing a decrease in pain. Because there is a widespread distribution of these receptors both inside and outside of the nervous system, opioid analgesics produce a wide spectrum of side effects. You can see euphoria, sedation, cardiovascular disorders such as a slow heart rate, respiratory depression, convulsion, nausea, vomiting, and itching.

A significant problem with opioid analgesics is the development of tolerance. The pain relief achieved lessens, so the tendency is to require higher and higher doses. Changing to a different medication can be beneficial, but practitioners need to have knowledge of proper conversion dosages. Pain management providers are an excellent resource for patients requiring chronic pain management with narcotics.

Excessive opioid exposure can produce a paradoxical increase in pain sensitivity. The biggest concern with chronic opioid use is addiction or misuse of medications. Addiction differs from physical dependence, which is commonly seen in individuals taking opioids over a prolonged period. Individuals experience physical withdrawal symptoms when they discontinue the opioid, demonstrating physical dependence. Tolerance is the term used to describe the need for increasing doses to maintain the same effect of pain relief. Addiction is a chronic, relapsing disorder that is characterized by drug-seeking behavior and continued use even when there are adverse consequences. With continued use, a person's ability to exert self-control can become seriously impaired.

Because of the current global opioid crisis, many practitioners are resistant to giving narcotic pain medications. Practitioners may preferentially use non-opioid alternatives. Narcotics should be used judiciously and with informed shared decision-making between the patient and their healthcare provider. Periodic follow-ups and monitoring for side effects, compliance, and effectiveness is important. Most patients will benefit from consultation with a pain management practitioner, who can help develop a plan for those with severe chronic pain.

Intravesical treatments

We refer to medications administered into the bladder as intravesical treatments or a bladder instillation. Medications are sometimes combined, in which case we call it a bladder cocktail. The medication is instilled into the bladder and then urinated out. Patients that have side effects from oral medications seem to better tolerate intravesical treatments. Patients with bladder-derived phenotypes or Ulcerative IC seem to benefit most from intravesical treatments. Patients with central sensitization syndrome, which is a brain-processing phenotype, may have an upregulation of C-fibers in the bladder wall and may benefit from bladder instillations. Instillations can help with IC/BPS flares in other phenotypes as well.

Clinicians can use a small 8 French pediatric catheter for the instillation to ease any discomfort from being catheterized. Using lidocaine jelly prior to the catheter insertion can also be helpful. Some patients are taught how to catheterize, so that they can do the instillations at home as needed. Having more control over the timing of the treatment alleviates some of the anxiety that some patients have about symptom flares.

Dimethyl Sulfoxide (DMSO) therapy is an FDA-approved intravesical treatment that is felt to have anti-inflammatory, analgesic, and muscle relaxant properties. Clinicians instill DMSO with a catheter. Patients hold it in the bladder for 15 minutes, and then urinate it out. It is typical to have a garlic-like taste and odor within a few minutes after the medication is put into the bladder. This odor on your breath and skin may last up to 72 hours. DMSO may increase absorption of other drugs, therefore it is often used in bladder cocktails with steroid medications (like hydrocortisone, Solu-Cortef, or triamcinolone), heparin, lidocaine, bupivacaine, and sodium bicarbonate to help these substances penetrate the bladder wall more easily.

Heparin is used as a bladder instillation to help reestablish the GAG layer. Studies have shown that when combined with alkalinized lidocaine, significant improvement can be achieved by certain individuals.

Lidocaine is a type of local anesthetic. It blocks pain signals arising from the nerve endings. Studies have shown that, as a bladder instillation, it significantly improves symptoms in the short term when compared to a placebo. When you make the solution more alkaline, the lidocaine penetrates the lining of the bladder better. In addition, when lidocaine is added to Elmiron® cocktails, or heparin, there appears to be a better improvement in symptoms compared to lidocaine alone.[63]

Sodium Hyaluronate (Cystistat®) is used to temporarily replace the GAG layer. It is not available in the US but is readily available in over 20 countries in Europe, Canada, and China.

Chondroitin sulfate (Uracyst® Hyacyst®) is a glycosaminoglycan (GAG) which temporarily replaces the GAG layer of the bladder and may have anti-inflammatory properties. It is not available in the US

---

63   Clemens JC, Erickson DR, Varela NP, and Lai HH: Diagnosis and treatment of interstitial cystitis/bladder pain syndrome. J. Urol 2022; 208: 34-42.

but is often used as a bladder instillation in Canada, Europe, China and many more countries. Studies have shown a decrease in IC/BPS symptoms with its use, with negligible side effects.

Procedures

Cystoscopy with hydrodistension is performed under anesthesia. Clinicians fill the bladder while monitoring pressure. We recommend clinicians use low-pressure hydrodistension (60-80 cm/H20) for a short duration (less than 10 minutes). The latest research suggests that hydrodistension is not mandatory to diagnose IC/BPS, yet it may still lead to positive outcomes. Hydrodistension will allow Hunner's ulcers or lesions to be identified, which then allows for treatment with fulguration and/or triamcinolone injection. Clinicians can take a biopsy if indicated, since they perform the procedure under anesthesia. Some patients find hydrodistension is therapeutic, with a noticeable improvement in IC/BPS symptoms. In addition, measuring the capacity of the bladder under anesthesia has a prognostic value. If an individual has a severely limited bladder capacity under anesthesia, it suggests a small fibrotic bladder, whereas a larger bladder capacity under anesthesia has a better prognosis. Treatments for IC/BPS may help with pain and urgency, but a small bladder may limit improvement in urinary frequency. A more normal anesthetic capacity carries a better prognosis, with IC/BPS treatments not only helping with pain and urgency but also improving the urinary frequency.

In a literature review by the American Urological Association (AUA), studies have shown clinical relief after hydrodistension ranging from 30-54 percent at one month, 18-56 percent at three months, and 0-7 percent at 5-6 months. Therefore, hydrodistension can be beneficial for some individuals, yet it may have to be performed repeatedly. Updated literature showed improvement in symptoms that ranged from 65 percent to greater than 90 percent at the 6-9-month follow-up. The AUA guidelines list cystoscopy with hydrodistension as an option.[64]

Botox® or onabotulinum toxin A (BTX-A) is not FDA-approved for the indication of IC/BPS. BTX-A is neurotoxic. If injected into a muscle, it will paralyze it, preventing it from contracting. It may also cause a desensitization in the nerves of the bladder, resulting in pain relief. Researchers have conducted clinical trials and injected BTX-A into the bladder, analyzing different areas for injections.

Injecting the bladder wall is a common treatment for those suffering from bladder spasms because of a neurological disorder like multiple sclerosis or spinal cord injury and for those with an overactive bladder. The risk of relaxing the bladder muscles too much is difficulty emptying the bladder or even not being able to urinate at all. If this were to occur, you would need to empty the bladder through intermittent catheterization. For patients with IC/BPS, studies have looked at injecting the BTX-A into the trigone, or the very bottom of the bladder, where many nerve endings converge. Injection of BTX-A into the trigone showed IC/BPS symptoms improved for up to 9-10 months, and there was no reported retention or need for catheterization.[65] The use of BTX-A, its mechanism of action in IC/BPS patients, the best location to inject, and the patient groups most likely to benefit are still being actively researched.

The second role for BTX-A is as an injection into the pelvic muscles or other affected muscles, when there is evidence of muscle spasms. This would be patients with the muscle/myofascial phenotype. Both single and repeat injections have shown a significant reduction in pain.[66] It is not clear what the mechanism of action is. It may be twofold.

64   Clemens JC, Erickson DR, Varela NP, and Lai HH: Diagnosis and treatment of interstitial cystitis/bladder pain syndrome. J. Urol 2022; 208: 34-42.

65   Pinto R, Lopes T, Silva J, et al: Persistent therapeutic effect of repeated injections of onabotulinum toxin A in refractory bladder pain syndrome/interstitial cystitis. J. Urol 2013; 189: 548.

66   Morrisey D, et al: Botulinum toxin A injections into pelvic floor muscles under electromyographic guidance for women with refractory high-tone pelvic floor dysfunction: A 6-month prospective pilot study. Female Pelvic Med. Reconstr. Surg 2015; 21(5): 277-82.

Patients may benefit from the relaxation of the muscle that is tense or spasming but may also benefit from a decrease in the nerve signals going to the brain that can cause pain and brain sensitization. Further research will help to clarify this.

Electrocautery and/or triamcinolone injection is a specific treatment done for individuals with Ulcerative Interstitial Cystitis phenotype with a Hunner's ulcer or lesion. We usually do the procedure under anesthesia. Sometimes, we may biopsy the lesion to confirm that no other pathology exists. Information about the type of inflammatory cells present can also help guide therapy. Fulguration is a way of "burning off" the lesion. Imagine creating a scab over the surface of the lesion. Both electrocautery and laser treatments can achieve this. It is possible to do fulguration alone, or together with a triamcinolone injection. Triamcinolone is a steroid which works as a potent anti-inflammatory agent. Patients can also have just the triamcinolone injection without fulguration.

Many patients with fulguration and/or triamcinolone injection alone will have symptom improvement. This has led to the recommendation by the AUA that fulguration and/or triamcinolone injection be used for Ulcerative Interstitial Cystitis to improve symptoms.[67] In one long-term study of 76 patients treated with fulguration by electrocautery, there was a significant improvement in pain, urgency, and frequency. 214 fulguration procedures were done. Overall, 89.6 percent of patients noted some improvement, 56.3 percent noted a marked improvement, and 84 percent of patients felt that the fulguration was the most beneficial treatment that they had received. The study also showed that even with multiple repeat fulgurations, there was no reduction in bladder capacity after single or multiple treatments.[68]

---

67   Clemens JC, Erickson DR, Varela NP, and Lai HH: Diagnosis and treatment of interstitial cystitis/bladder pain syndrome. J. Urol 2022; 208: 34-42.

68   Chennamsetty A, Khourdaji I, Goike J, et al: Electrosurgical management of Hunner's ulcers in a referral center's interstitial cystitis population. Urol 2015; 85(10): 74-8.

Triamcinolone injection alone has been used as well. One study in patients with ulcers showed a 70 percent improvement in symptoms with an average duration of improvement of 7-12 months.[69] I have found triamcinolone injection alone to be beneficial for patients that can tolerate it with local anesthesia in the office. This prevents a trip to the OR and anesthesia.

Neuromodulation with implantation involves the stimulation of nerves via an electrical device implanted into the patient. Using neuromodulation is still considered experimental for pain. Sacral nerve neuromodulation is FDA-approved for retention, urgency/frequency, urge incontinence, and fecal incontinence. Interstim® has been FDA-approved since 1997. Since then, they have approved other devices, such as Axonics®. Sacral neuromodulation has been useful in refractory IC/BPS patients with a decrease in frequency, hesitancy, and a decrease in narcotic medication use.[70] In a recent study, patients with IC/BPS were found to have a 65 percent improvement in urinary urgency, frequency, nighttime voiding, and an improvement in bladder volume, with a median follow-up of 20.1, plus or minus 12.8 months.[71]

An advantage of neuromodulation is that clinicians can place an electrode for a test and trial it for a couple of weeks. They typically place the electrode for this test with local anesthetic and sedation. You can experience what the neuromodulation sensation feels like, and you can see if it improves your symptoms prior to committing to the implantation of the neurostimulator. This allows you to test drive the stimulation. You can also stimulate the pudendal nerve instead of a sacral nerve.

---

69   Cox M, Klutke JJ, and Klutke CG: Assessment of patient outcomes following submucosal injection of triamcinolone for treatment of Hunner's ulcer subtype of interstitial cystitis. Can. J. Urol 2009; 16(2): 4536-40.

70   Peters KM, Konstant D: Sacral neuromodulation decreases narcotic requirements in refractory interstitial cystitis. BJU 2004; 93(6): 777-779.

71   Zhang P, Wang JY, Zhang Y, et al: Results of sacral neuromodulation therapy for urinary voiding dysfunction: Five-year experience of a retrospective, multicenter study in China. Neuromodulation 2019; 22: 730.

In another study, patients were tested with sacral nerve stimulation and pudendal nerve stimulation at separate times. Patients could then select the test that provided the best improvement in their symptoms. Based on the test that they preferred, they either had a sacral or a pudendal neurostimulator placed. At six months post-implantation of the neurostimulator, 66 percent of patients that chose the pudendal nerve implant had greater symptom relief than those patients who chose the sacral nerve implants. Stimulating the pudendal nerve via neuromodulation has also been beneficial for those with pudendal neuralgia or the neuralgia phenotype.

Newer stimulators last longer, some are rechargeable, and some are MRI-compatible. The size of the implants has also gotten much smaller. There are side effects and complications associated with neuromodulation, including mechanical malfunction and radiation of the stimulation to the leg or pain at the implant or lead site. Infections can occur, requiring removal of the neuromodulation system. As with any surgical procedure, all risks and benefits need to be considered when choosing to have an implant placed.

The AUA lists neuromodulation as an option for treatment when other treatments have not provided adequate symptom control and quality-of-life improvement.[72]

Transcutaneous electrical nerve stimulation or TENS therapy has been used with success in some individuals. TENS therapy carries negligible risk. TENS is a treatment used for pain relief that uses a mild electrical current applied to the skin. A TENS machine is a small battery-operated device which attaches to leads which are connected to sticky pads called electrodes. You attach electrodes to the skin, commonly in the suprapubic area and lower back. The machine then sends small electrical impulses to the area, which you will feel as a tingling sensation.

---

72   Clemens JC, Erickson DR, Varela NP, and Lai HH: Diagnosis and treatment of interstitial cystitis/bladder pain syndrome. J Urol 2022; 208: 34-42.

The electrical impulses from the TENS unit can reduce the pain signals going to the spinal cord and the brain. Researchers have shown the electrical signal to help relieve pain and relax muscles for some individuals. There is some thought that the signals may also stimulate the production of endorphins, which are the body's natural painkillers. Physical therapists will sometimes be able to do a test with a TENS unit to see if this helps with your symptoms of pain. There are few risks, but some will be sensitive to the adhesive on the pads. Patients should not use a TENS unit if you have a pacemaker or other neurostimulator. There is sparse literature on the use of TENS for patients with IC/BPS.

Percutaneous tibial nerve stimulation or PTNS involves the placement of a small acupuncture needle into the area of the posterior tibial nerve near your ankle. An electrical signal goes through the needle, and patients typically feel a sensation going down towards the big toe. The stimulation should not be painful. Clinicians administer electrical signals for 30 minutes, usually weekly for 12 weeks. Clinicians perform PTNS in the office, and it is FDA-approved for frequency, urgency, and urge incontinence. There is sparse literature for treatment of IC/BPS, and the literature that exists has shown conflicting results. We need to conduct more research to determine if specific subtypes of IC/BPS patients may benefit from PTNS. Patients with overlapping symptoms of overactive bladder may show some benefit. Studies have shown 71-80 percent success in patients with overactive bladder.[73]

Pudendal nerve block is a procedure where an anesthetic and sometimes a steroid is injected into the area around the pudendal nerve. This blocks nerve impulses coming from the nerve. This may be done with X-ray or ultrasound guidance and can be performed through the vagina or the buttocks (transgluteally). If you have improvement in pain after a pudendal nerve block, then it would be likely that the pudendal nerve is involved in your pain, consistent with a neuralgia

---

73   Govier FE, Litwiller S, Nitti V, Kreder KJ, Rosenblatt P: Percutaneous afferent neuromodulation for the refractory overactive bladder: results of a multicenter study. J. Urol 2001; 165(4): 1193-8.

phenotype. A pudendal nerve block is used to help diagnose the neuralgia phenotype, specifically pudendal neuralgia. Repeating the injections can eliminate or reduce the pain for many patients. Patients with pudendal neuralgia will usually get symptom relief with a pudendal nerve block, especially when a multidisciplinary approach is used to treat their symptoms.[74]

Potential risks and side effects are minimal, and serious complications are rare. Risks include new or increased pain, infection, bleeding, skin change, allergic or unexpected drug reaction, or unintended nerve injury.

Trigger point injections involve injection of an anesthetic into discrete myofascial trigger points for immediate relief and a corticosteroid for more sustained relief. Trigger point injections are usually combined with pelvic floor physical therapy for individuals with a muscle/myofascial phenotype. This treatment may arrest the neurogenic triggers that can lead to bladder symptoms and may decrease the central nervous system sensitivity that contributes to pain from the dysfunctional muscles.[75]

Healthcare providers can palpate and inject trigger points in the abdominal wall directly. Trigger points in the pelvic floor muscles are approached vaginally in women, whereas men may have injections through the rectum or the perineum. One study in men with chronic pelvic pain syndrome showed improvement in about one-half of patients when trigger point injection was combined with pelvic floor physical therapy.[76]

Acupuncture involves the insertion of very thin needles through the skin at strategic points on the body. Acupuncture has long been

---

74   Gupta P, Gaines N, Sirls L, Peters KM: A multidisciplinary approach to the evaluation and treatment of interstitial cystitis/bladder pain syndrome: An ideal model of care. Transl. Androl. Urol 2015; 4(6): 611-19.

75   Weiss JM: Pelvic floor myofascial trigger points: Manual therapy for interstitial cystitis and the urgency-frequency syndrome. J. Urol 2001; 166: 2200-31.

76   Tadros NN, et al: Utility of trigger point injection as an adjunct to physical therapy in men with chronic prostatitis/chronic pain syndrome. Trans. Androl. Urol 2017; 6(3): 534-7.

a key component of traditional Chinese medicine. Eastern medicine practitioners believe that acupuncture can restore balance to the body's energy, referred to as chi. These energy pathways are called meridians and run through the body. Practitioners insert needles into specific meridians with the goal of regaining balance. Western medicine views acupuncture points as areas where certain nerves, muscles, or tissue can be activated. Some believe that this stimulation can boost your body's natural endorphins or painkillers. The risk of acupuncture is low. Common side effects include soreness and minor bruising or bleeding at the site of the needle insertion.

There have been studies looking at the role of acupuncture in pelvic pain in both men and women, with evidence that this treatment may benefit some patients.[77]

In one study of 440 men with chronic prostatitis/chronic pelvic pain, men were randomized into either a treatment group that received 20 sessions of acupuncture over eight weeks or a sham group. There was significant improvement in symptoms of pain, voiding dysfunction, anxiety, depression, and quality of life that lasted up to 24 weeks after the treatment. There was a positive response rate of 60.5 percent seen in the treatment group compared to 36.8 percent in the sham group at eight weeks. The results were durable over time.[78]

Acupuncture has also been beneficial for some patients with myofascial syndrome not responsive to local anesthetic blocks. The researchers performed acupuncture at abdominal wall trigger points once a week for 10 weeks. Results showed a significant decrease in pain intensity, and patients had sustained effects at six months.[79] This

77   Giray Sonmez M, Kozanhan B: Complete response to acupuncture therapy in female patients with refractory interstitial cystitis/bladder pain syndrome. Ginekol Pol 2017; 88(2): 61-67.

78   Sun Y, et al: Acupuncture improved chronic prostatitis/chronic pelvic pain syndrome symptoms. Ann. Int. Med. 2021; doi: 10.7326/M21-1814.

79   Mitidieri AM, Gurian MB, et al: Effect of acupuncture on chronic pelvic pain secondary to abdominal myofascial syndrome not responsive to local anesthetic block: a pilot study. Med. Acupunct 2017; 29(6): 397-404.

complementary therapy is still being researched and may hold promise for certain subgroups of patients.

Additional alternative therapies

Medical Marijuana/CBD is becoming more readily available as more states have legalized the use of medical marijuana. As of 2023, 38 states, three territories, and the District of Columbia allow the medical use of cannabis products. The endocannabinoid system is involved in pain perception and inflammation. Cannabis contains delta-9-tetrahydrocannabinol (THC) and cannabidiol (CBD). The psychoactive cannabinoid THC can bring about a 'high' feeling. Using THC stimulates appetite, reduces PTSD symptoms, and aids sleep. CBD (the non-psychoactive cannabinoid) reduces inflammation, relieves anxiety, and reduces seizures. The combination of THC and CBD may act as a muscle relaxant, relieve spasms, reduce nausea, and relieve pain.

In one large review of the literature looking at the use of medical cannabis for gynecologic pain conditions, of which IC/BPS was included, most women reported that cannabis improved pain.[80] Unfortunately, there is sparse literature specifically addressing the use of medical marijuana for IC/BPS.

Dr. J Curtis Nickel published a review of the use of medical marijuana for chronic pelvic pain in 2018.[81] He thought there were seven lessons to be learned about medical cannabis.

1. That basic research supports the theoretical use of medical marijuana.
2. That there was limited research to provide strong support for its use in urologic chronic pelvic pain syndromes.

80 Liang AL, Gingher EL, Coleman JS: Medical cannabis for gynecologic pain conditions: A systematic review. Obstet. Gynecol 2022; 139(2): 287-296.

81 Nickel JC. Medical marijuana for urologic chronic pelvic pain. Can. Urol. Assoc. J 2018; 12(6 Suppl 3): S181-S183.

3. That marijuana was better than opioids.
4. That some high-risk patients should not be prescribed medical marijuana, for example, if there is a history of substance abuse, diversion risk, or mood disorders.
5. Patient education is the key to successful use of medical marijuana.
6. Dosing considerations are necessary. One should "start low and go slow."
7. Patient follow-up is mandatory.

Literature suggests that marijuana can reduce pain by 37 percent.

To understand how medical marijuana works, you must first understand the complicated pain transmission pathway. We can break the pain transmission pathway down into three steps. The first step involves when the pain-sensing cells, for example, in the muscles or the bladder, become stimulated. The second step involves the transmission of those signals up the spinal cord to the brain. The third step involves the brain, which then must interpret the signal it receives.

Patients with chronic pain often perceive these signals that the brain receives as pain. It is felt that cannabinoids may affect the periphery (i.e., the bladder and muscles) by preventing activation of the pain-sensing neurons. It may also affect the brain, and how it perceives the signal. We need more research to fully understand how cannabinoids work in patients with chronic pain.

Side effects of medical marijuana can include dizziness, nausea, fatigue, sleepiness, euphoria, vomiting, disorientation, confusion, loss of balance, and hallucinations.

Topical anesthetics such as lidocaine 5 percent patches. A lidocaine 5 percent patch is a prescription medication that is used to treat symptoms of nerve pain or neuralgia and for the temporary relief of pain. Clinicians may use a lidocaine 5 percent patch alone or in combination with other medications. I have found that this has been useful for some patients during a flare and may be beneficial for those with myofascial pain syndrome with abdominal trigger points or tenderness. Patients with neuralgia phenotype may benefit from a lidocaine 5 percent patch as well. Patients can place the patch in the suprapubic area, once for up to 12 hours in a 24-hour period. Side effects can include burning at the site of application, stinging, irritation, sudden dizziness or drowsiness after application, confusion, blurred vision, ringing in your ears, and unusual sensations of temperature. Over-the-counter lidocaine 4 percent patches are also available now.

Compounded drugs: Drug compounding is usually regarded as combining, mixing, or altering ingredients to create a medication tailored to the unique needs of an individual. A compounding pharmacist can create oral, topical, instillation, or suppository medications. The FDA has not approved compounded drugs. For a patient who cannot be treated with an FDA-approved medication, a drug can be created specifically for them, such as someone with an allergy to a certain dye who requires a medication without it. They may make compounded drugs for a different delivery method, for example, a liquid version for someone who cannot swallow a pill. In addition, unique combinations of medications can be formulated that are not otherwise available, as in the topical creams often used to treat vulvodynia or the urethral phenotype.

Diazepam or Valium®: A commonly used compounded drug for patients with IC/BPS is vaginal or rectal diazepam or Valium®. This suppository offers an alternative way to take diazepam, which is used as a muscle relaxant and may have fewer side effects than taking it orally. Patients with myofascial pain syndrome or pelvic floor dysfunction may use a diazepam vaginal or rectal suppository either alone or with the addition of baclofen, lidocaine, ketamine, or amitriptyline. The suppositories help to relax the muscles of the pelvic floor. Patients with the urethral phenotype may also benefit from Valium® suppositories.

Vulvodynia creams: Patients with vulvodynia may benefit from a topical compounded cream. Compounding pharmacists typically make the cream pH-balanced, without preservatives or alcohol that can create symptoms. There are many formulations that may include topical gabapentin, ketamine, amitriptyline, baclofen, cyclobenzaprine, and lidocaine. These creams are also helpful for those with the urethral phenotype.

Some patients benefit from compounded estrogen creams to treat the genitourinary syndrome of menopause, especially if they need a preservative-free formulation because of allergies.

Low-dose naltrexone (LDN) is an off-label, compounded drug that has been used with chronic pain. Clinicians typically prescribe naltrexone for opioid dependence or alcohol dependence. Research has shown a decrease in symptom intensity for Crohn's disease, multiple sclerosis, fibromyalgia, and complex regional pain syndrome. It has been hypothesized that low-dose naltrexone might operate as an anti-inflammatory agent in the central nervous system, via action on microglial cells. Researchers are currently exploring the possibility of treating long COVID with a low dose of naltrexone.

Given the limited research, the use of LDN for chronic pain is still considered experimental. As a daily oral medication, it is inexpensive and well-tolerated. You cannot combine it with opioid medications. We need clinical trials to help understand how LDN works, and which patients will benefit most. LDN could be one of the first glial cell modulators used to manage chronic pain disorders.

Chapter 25

Final Thoughts

As I have alluded to throughout this book, this is a very exciting time for patients with IC/BPS. The "Multidisciplinary Approach to the Study of Chronic Pelvic Pain" (MAPP) Research Network was established by the NIDDK to better understand the pathophysiology of urologic chronic pelvic pain syndromes. The goal is to help direct future clinical trials and improve clinical care (www.mappnetwork. org). There have been tremendous strides made in the understanding of IC/BPS phenotyping and capturing some of the differences between the subgroups or phenotypes of patients.

In an interesting publication looking at IC/BPS and associated medical conditions, with an emphasis on IBS, fibromyalgia, and chronic fatigue syndrome, another concept was brought up.[82] It is possible to have **organ-centric pain** symptoms, involving only the bladder, the bowel, or the vagina (think bladder-derived BPS or Ulcerative IC, IBS, or vulvodynia). Over time, pain may become more regional, affecting surrounding areas (**regional pain syndrome**). It is possible

---

82   Nickel JC, Tripp DA, Pontari M, Moldwin R, et al: Interstitial cystitis/painful bladder syndrome and associated medical conditions with an emphasis on irritable bowel syndrome, fibromyalgia, and chronic fatigue syndrome.
J. Urol 2010; 184: 1358-1363.

to start with IC/BPS focused on the bladder and then become more regional and include IBS or vice versa. In this study 38.6 percent of IC/BPS patients had IBS compared to 5.2 percent in the control group. It is then possible to develop a more **systemic pain syndrome** such as fibromyalgia or chronic fatigue syndrome. Fibromyalgia was seen in 17.7 percent of IC/BPS patients versus 2.6 percent of controls, and chronic fatigue syndrome was seen in 9.5 percent of IC/BPS patients versus 1.7 percent of controls. As the number of associated conditions increased—i.e., going from organ-centric to regional to systemic—stress, pain, depression, and sleep disturbances increased while quality of life decreased. Clearly, more longitudinal studies need to be completed to see if this is a progression that occurs over time as well as the impact on clinical therapy.

Phenotypes are constantly being researched with the goal of directing research and ultimately therapy. There is ongoing research into the brain's function, and changes that may help guide therapy for the brain-processing phenotype. It truly is an exciting time, with a tremendous amount of research ongoing.

Toolbox

- Bladder Diary
- Bladder Retraining
- Questionnaires
- Physiological quieting exercises
- Resources

Bladder Diary

IC Journey to Wellness
Interstitial Cystitis and Bladder Pain Syndrome

Fluid Intake	Time	Output	Notes: urgency, pain, leakage etc

Total fluids in=_____ | Average bladder capacity: Day:_____ Night:_____

Bladder Retraining

The goal of bladder retraining is to increase bladder capacity, which will then result in less frequency of urination, both day and night. Over time, when you urinate often, before the bladder has reached its normal capacity, the bladder will shrink and get smaller. The result is more frequency, as the bladder holds less. With IC/BPS, frequency is common, as there is discomfort as the bladder fills. Once the pain or discomfort has improved with treatment of the IC/BPS, the frequency will often continue because the bladder has gotten smaller. The good news is that in most cases, you can stretch the bladder back out to a more normal size, which will then improve the frequency of urination.

So how do you accomplish that? Slowly, you can increase your bladder capacity. The goal is to go gradually, to not cause a flare of symptoms from over-distending the bladder too quickly.

Take a disposable cup and urinate a comfortably full bladder into the cup, then draw a line and mark the date on the cup. It may only be a few ounces at the beginning. Over the next month, when you get the first urge to urinate, try to distract yourself. Read a few more emails, wait until the next set of commercials on the TV, or read one more chapter in your book. Try to wait 5-10 minutes and then go to the bathroom. Do not wait until you are in pain. Just try to postpone urination for at least five more minutes. One month later, pull out the cup, and urinate a full bladder into the cup. You should notice the line is a little higher than what you recorded previously. Slowly, the bladder capacity will increase, and the line on the cup will continue to rise higher and higher.

Some patients will measure the volume and keep a chart. The easiest is to just keep the same cup and celebrate as the line climbs up the cup. As your bladder capacity increases, slowly, you will notice you are getting up less at night and urinating less during the day.

The key is to go slow. Adequate hydration is important. It is easier to do this if you are drinking fluids during the day. I have seen patients go from tiny three-ounce bladders up to almost normal-sized bladders.

Another bad habit that patients with IC/BPS have is to urinate before they leave the house, just in case. Patients with IC/BPS often urinate to prevent pain or discomfort, which often leads to toilet mapping. To put it simply, you know where the bathrooms are everywhere! Try not to urinate "just in case." Only urinate when you really must go. Put off going to the bathroom for five minutes when you feel the need to go. This will allow the bladder to fill a little fuller, and slowly, it will get bigger. Remember, bladder retraining should not cause significant pain or leakage. If you are getting uncomfortable, then urinate. Bladder retraining is easiest to do when you know the bathroom is nearby. Therefore, there is no anxiety produced as you know you can urinate if you need to.

Patients should address the symptoms of pain and pressure before attempting bladder retraining. The frequency is usually the last to improve with therapy for IC/BPS because of the bladder getting smaller over time. It takes time to stretch it back out to a more normal size. Be patient and celebrate each time the line goes up, even a little, on that cup!

Questionnaires

Some of the questionnaires discussed at the beginning of the book have been included. You can do the questionnaires at the beginning of your journey, and then you can repeat them after therapy. Ideally, if therapy is having a positive effect on your symptoms, scores should show an improvement. The questionnaires provided have all been validated as good measures of patient-reported symptoms. It may feel like you are not getting better, as the changes to your symptoms can be subtle and slow to occur. When the questionnaires and the bladder diary are repeated, there are often objective improvements seen that you may not have even noticed. A lowering of your scores will show that improvement is being made. Be patient and recheck periodically to see the changes. Celebrate the lower scores, realizing that you are moving in the right direction.

These questionnaires are often used in clinical studies to assess improvement in symptoms. They are not used solely for diagnostic purposes. They are at times combined with clinical history and clinical exam findings to aid in diagnosis.

You can access all the questionnaires discussed at https://icjourneytowellness.com or by scanning:

QUEENSLAND FEMALE PELVIC FLOOR QUESTIONNAIRE

Incomplete bowel evacuation Do have the feeling of incomplete bowel emptying?	**Obstructed defecation** Do you use finger pressure to help empty your bowel?	**How much of a bother** is your bowel problem to you?
0 never	0 never	0 no problem
1 occasionally – < 1/week	1 occasionally – < 1/week	1 slightly
2 frequently -> 1/week	2 frequently -> 1/week	2 moderately
3 daily	3 daily	3 greatly
Other symptoms (pain, mucous discharge, rectal prolapse etc.)		

Prolapse section Q27 –31 Score _____ / 15 = _____

Prolapse sensation Do you get a sensation of tissue protrusion in your vagina/lump/bulging?	**Vaginal pressure or heaviness** Do you experience vag. pressure/ heaviness/dragging sensation?	**Prolapse reduction to void** Do you have to push back your prolapse in order to void?
0 never	0 never	0 never
1 occasionally – < 1/week	1 occasionally – < 1/week	1 occasionally – < 1/week
2 frequently -> 1/week	2 frequently -> 1/week	2 frequently -> 1/week
3 daily	3 daily	3 daily
Prolapse reduction to defaecate Do you have to push back your prolapse to empty your bowels?	**How much of a bother** is the prolapse to you?	
0 never		
1 occasionally – < 1/week	0 no problem	
2 frequently -> 1/week	1 slightly	
3 daily	2 moderately	
	3 greatly	
Other symptoms (problems sitting/walking, pain, vag. bleeding)		

Sexual function Section Q 32 – Score _____ / 19

Sexually active? Are you sexually active?	**If NOT, why not:**	**Sufficient lubrication** Do you have sufficient lubrication during intercourse?
no	no partner	1 no
< 1/week	partner unable	0 yes
≥ 1/week	vaginal dryness	
most days / daily	too painful Prolapse ⎫ 19	
	embarrassment Prolapse ⎭	
	other	
During intercourse vaginal sensation is:	**Vaginal laxity** Do you feel that your vagina is too loose or lax?	**Vaginal tightness/vaginismus** Do you feel that your vagina is too tight?
3 none	0 never	0 never
3 painful	1 occasionally	1 occasionally
1 minimal	2 frequently	2 frequently
0 normal / pleasant	3 always	3 always
Dyspareunia Do you experience pain with intercourse:	**Dyspareunia where** Where does the pain occur	**Coital incontinence** Do you leak urine during sex?
0 never	no pain	0 never
1 occasionally	at the entrance of the vagina	1 occasionally
2 frequently	deep inside/ in the pelvis	2 frequently
3 always	both	3 always
How much of a bother are these sexual issues to you? Not applicable	**Other symptoms** (coital flatus or faecal incontinence, vaginismus etc.)	
0 no problem at all		
1 slight problem		
2 moderate problem		
3 great problem		

TOTAL Pelvic floor Dysfunction SCORE:_____

Reference: Baessler K, O'Neill SM, Maher CF, Battistutta D. A validated self-administered female pelvic floor questionnaire. Int Urogynecol J. 2010 Feb; 21(2):163-72.

INTERNATIONAL PROSTATE SYMPTOM SCORE (I-PSS)

Patient Name: Date:	Not At All	Less Than 1 Time In 5	Less Than Half The Time	About Half The Time	More Than Half The Time	Almost Always	YOUR SCORE
1. Incomplete Emptying Over the past month, how often have you had a sensation of not emptying your bladder completely after you finish urinating?	0	1	2	3	4	5	
2. Frequency Over the past month, how often have you had to urinate again less than two hours after you have finished urinating?	0	1	2	3	4	5	
3. Intermittency Over the past month, how often have you found you stopped and started again several times when you urinated?	0	1	2	3	4	5	
4. Urgency Over the past month, how often have you found it difficult to postpone urination?	0	1	2	3	4	5	
5. Weak Stream Over the last month, how often have you had a weak urinary stream?	0	1	2	3	4	5	
6. Straining Over the past month, how often have you had to push or strain to begin urination?	0	1	2	3	4	5	

	None	Once	Twice	3 times	4 times	5 or more	YOUR SCORE
7. Nocturia Over the past month how many times did you most typically get up each night to urinate from the time you went to bed until the time you got up in the morning?	0	1	2	3	4	5	
Total I-PSS Score							

Quality of Life due to Urinary Symptoms	Delighted	Pleased	Mostly satisfied	Mixed	Mostly unhappy	Unhappy	Terrible
If you were to spend the rest of your life with your urinary condition just the way it is now, how would you feel about that?	0	1	2	3	4	5	6

The I-PSS is based on the answers to seven questions concerning urinary symptoms. Each question is assigned points from 0 to 5 indicating increasing severity of the particular symptom. The total score can therefore range from 0 to 35 (asymptomatic to very symptomatic).

Although there are presently no standard recommendations into grading patients with mild, moderate or severe symptoms, patients can be tentatively classified as follows: **0 - 7 = mildly symptomatic; 8 - 19 = moderately symptomatic; 20 - 35 = severely symptomatic.**

The International Consensus Committee (ICC) recommends the use of only a single question to assess the patient's quality of life. The answers to this question range from "delighted" to "terrible" or 0 to 6. Although this single question may or may not capture the global impact of BPH symptoms on quality of life, it may serve as a valuable starting point for doctor-patient conversation.

Reference: Barry MJ, Fowler FJ, O'Leary MP, Bruskewitz RC, Holtgrewe HL, Mebust WK, et al. The American Urological Association Symptom Index for benign prostatic hyperplasia. J Urol 1992; 148(5):1549-1557.

CENTRAL SENSITIZATION INVENTORY: PART A

Name: _____   Date: _____

Please circle the best response to the right of each statement.

1	I feel tired and unrefreshed when I wake from sleeping.	Never	Rarely	Sometimes	Often	Always
2	My muscles feel stiff and achy.	Never	Rarely	Sometimes	Often	Always
3	I have anxiety attacks.	Never	Rarely	Sometimes	Often	Always
4	I grind or clench my teeth.	Never	Rarely	Sometimes	Often	Always
5	I have problems with diarrhea and/or constipation.	Never	Rarely	Sometimes	Often	Always
6	I need help in performing my daily activities.	Never	Rarely	Sometimes	Often	Always
7	I am sensitive to bright lights.	Never	Rarely	Sometimes	Often	Always
8	I get tired very easily when I am physically active.	Never	Rarely	Sometimes	Often	Always
9	I feel pain all over my body.	Never	Rarely	Sometimes	Often	Always
10	I have headaches.	Never	Rarely	Sometimes	Often	Always
11	I feel discomfort in my bladder and/or burning when I urinate.	Never	Rarely	Sometimes	Often	Always
12	I do not sleep well.	Never	Rarely	Sometimes	Often	Always
13	I have difficulty concentrating.	Never	Rarely	Sometimes	Often	Always
14	I have skin problems such as dryness, itchiness, or rashes.	Never	Rarely	Sometimes	Often	Always
15	Stress makes my physical symptoms get worse.	Never	Rarely	Sometimes	Often	Always
16	I feel sad or depressed.	Never	Rarely	Sometimes	Often	Always
17	I have low energy.	Never	Rarely	Sometimes	Often	Always
18	I have muscle tension in my neck and shoulders.	Never	Rarely	Sometimes	Often	Always
19	I have pain in my jaw.	Never	Rarely	Sometimes	Often	Always
20	Certain smells, such as perfumes, make me feel dizzy and nauseated.	Never	Rarely	Sometimes	Often	Always
21	I have to urinate frequently.	Never	Rarely	Sometimes	Often	Always
22	My legs feel uncomfortable and restless when I am trying to go to sleep at night.	Never	Rarely	Sometimes	Often	Always
23	I have difficulty remembering things.	Never	Rarely	Sometimes	Often	Always
24	I suffered trauma as a child.	Never	Rarely	Sometimes	Often	Always
25	I have pain in my pelvic area.	Never	Rarely	Sometimes	Often	Always

Total=

Reference: Neblett R. (2018). The Central Sensitization Inventory: A User's Manual. *Journal of Applied Biobehavioral Research*. 23(2):e12123

CENTRAL SENSITIZATION INVENTORY: PART B

Name: _____

Date: _____

Have you been diagnosed by a doctor with any of the following disorders?

Please check the box to the right for each diagnosis and write the year of the diagnosis.

		NO	YES	Year Diagnosed
1	Restless Leg Syndrome			
2	Chronic Fatigue Syndrome			
3	Fibromyalgia			
4	Temporomandibular Joint Disorder (TMJ)			
5	Migraine or tension headaches			
6	Irritable Bowel Syndrome			
7	Multiple Chemical Sensitivities			
8	Neck Injury (including whiplash)			
9	Anxiety or Panic Attacks			
10	Depression			

Physiological Quieting Techniques

Our nervous system gets wound up with the busyness of our lives, and with the stress of dealing with a chronic illness such as IC/BPS. This causes an increased outflow of nerve signals from the nervous system, which will often worsen symptoms. You can practice simple techniques to quiet the nervous system and improve symptoms.

A remarkably simple technique is deep breathing. Many smartphones have an app that will help guide you through simple breathing exercises. Try to do these several times a day. You do not need an app on the phone to do deep breathing, however. Simply take a deep breath, inhaling through your nose and exhaling through your mouth. Focus on the sensation of your breath as it moves in and out of your body. Try going slowly, inhaling to a count of five and then slowly exhaling. Try to relax and visualize the waves rolling in from the ocean. As the waves roll in, inhale. Then as the wave rolls out, exhale.

Diaphragmatic breathing is also called abdominal breathing or deep breathing. It is a relaxation technique that involves focusing on the movement of the diaphragm while breathing. It can help reduce stress, promote relaxation, and improve oxygen exchange in the body. To do diaphragmatic breathing, follow these steps:

1. Find a comfortable position, ideally a quiet place where you can sit or lie down, whichever is more comfortable for you.

2. Place your hand on your abdomen, just above your belly button, and the other on your chest. This will help you feel the movement of your breath.

3. Inhale slowly: Inhale slowly through your nose. As you inhale, focus on allowing your abdomen to rise. You should feel your hand on your abdomen moving outward while the hand on your chest remains relatively still.

4. Exhale gradually: Exhale slowly and completely through your mouth. As you exhale, your abdomen should naturally fall back down. Focus on making your exhale longer than your inhale to assist with calming.

5. Repeat: Continue this process of slow, deep breaths for several minutes. Try to maintain a steady and rhythmic breathing pattern.

6. Focus on the breath: While practicing diaphragmatic breathing, you can choose to focus your attention on your breath itself or use a calming word or phrase as a mantra. This can help keep your mind centered and prevent it from wandering.

7. Practice regularly: Diaphragmatic breathing is most effective when practiced regularly. You can incorporate it into your daily routine, such as during moments of stress, before sleep, or as part of a relaxation exercise.

Muscle relaxation is another technique that is very useful for patients with IC/BPS. Start at the top of your body and relax the muscles in your face and jaw, then drift down to your neck, shoulders, arm, fingers. Keep on going and relax your abdomen, hips, legs, calves, ankles, and toes. Slowly, move and relax each muscle as you move down. Picture yourself going limp; try to take your time and focus on each muscle as you sequentially relax your way down the body. This is nice to do when you are ready for bed, or any time you feel yourself tensing up. Try doing your breathing exercises at the same time, and visualize your happy place—the woods, the park, the beach, a comfy hammock swaying in the breeze.

Mindful meditation is a practice you should try to do daily. Focus on the present. Do not worry about the future or dwell on the past. Take a few moments to reflect on what you are grateful for. Notice the good things in life and work towards an appreciation for them. Go for a walk, ideally in a natural environment. Research has shown that nature has a lot to offer us, with positive benefits just being outside around the trees, the grass, the flowers. Notice the sounds, smells, and sensations around you. This helps to take the focus off the bladder and onto positive things that are right in front of us that we often don't appreciate.

Yoga is a wonderful way to relax and be in the moment. Yoga can be done in a class or in the comfort of your home. There are many online yoga classes available on YouTube. Just search for gentle yoga. Most yoga exercises will start with deep breathing and relaxation. Continue with mild stretching poses such as the child pose. Try to sit and let your legs fall to the side like a butterfly. Lying on your back, you can bend your legs, then pull them up towards your shoulders. Even a few minutes of yoga stretches can help quiet the nervous system and gently stretch your muscles. I have included some excellent resources, written by physical therapists, with stretches that will help the pelvic muscles relax and aid in overall quieting of the nervous system.

Visualization or **guided imagery** is a terrific way to quiet the nervous system. Visualize yourself in a tranquil environment, such as reclining on a hammock and admiring the clouds, at the shore with the pleasant sunshine and enchanting sound of the surf, or in the woodlands, with the breeze stirring through the branches, birds singing. Focus on the environment, the sounds, the feeling of the breeze on your skin. Transport yourself to your happy place. Any time that your symptoms are getting out of control, close your eyes and try to put yourself in that place. Breathe and just go there.

Resources

Interstitial Cystitis Association: www.ichelp.org

IC Network: www.ic-network.com

Both organizations above have up-to-date resources for patients with IC/BPS, including lists of providers that care for patients, diet information, support group listings, and much more. If you have not yet checked them out, I highly recommend it!

Additional Online Resources:

International Pelvic Pain Society- www.pelvicpain.org

American Urologic Association (AUA)- www.urologyhealth.org

International Painful Bladder Foundation- www.painful-bladder.org

European Society for the Study of BPS- www.essic.org

National Kidney and Urologic Diseases (NIDDK)- www.kidney.niddk.nih.gov

Multidisciplinary Approach to the Study of Chronic Pelvic Pain- www.mappnetwork.org

The IC Diet Project: Low-Acid Eating Made Simple- www.icdietproject.com

Books to consider:

There are many books that focus on dealing with IC/BPS or living with chronic pain. This list is by no means inclusive.

Interstitial Cystitis/Bladder Pain Syndrome and Chronic Pain
IC 101, by Gaye Grissom Sandler, Jill Heidi Osborne, MA, and Andrew B Sandler PhD (2021)

- Published in 2021, this is an up-to-date look at IC/BPS, with excellent self-help ideas and resources. *IC 101* introduces the concept of phenotyping IC/BPS.

The Interstitial Cystitis Solution: A Holistic Plan for Healing Painful Symptoms, Resolving Bladder and Pelvic Floor Dysfunction, and Taking Back your Life, by Nicole Cozean and Jesse Cozean (2016)

- Covers topics such as diet and nutrition, natural supplements, stress management, pelvic floor exercises, and excellent stretching routines.

You Are Not Your Pain: Using Mindfulness to Relieve Pain, Reduce Stress, and Restore Well-Being—an Eight-week Program, by Vidyamala Burch and Danny Penman (2015)

-This book offers an eight-week mindfulness-based program with eight audio meditations. These mindfulness-based practices soothe the brain's network.

Secret Suffering: How Women's Sexual and Pelvic Pain Affects Their Relationships, by Susan Bilheimer and Dr. Robert J. Echenberg (2019)

-Written by a gynecologist and leader in pelvic pain, this book discusses chronic pelvic and sexual pain, providing a blueprint for regaining intimacy in your relationships and managing chronic pelvic pain.

The Trigger Point Therapy Workbook—Your Self-Treatment Guide for Pain Relief by Clair Davies, NCTMB, and Amber Davies, NCTMB, LMT, et al. (2013)

-Excellent resource for those with muscle/myofascial phenotype

The Interstitial Cystitis Survival Guide, by Robert M. Moldwin, M.D., FACS (2000)

-Although published in 2000, still has excellent self-help advice that is pertinent today.

Interstitial Cystitis and Pain—Taking Control—A Handbook for People with IC and Their Caregivers, Published by the Interstitial Cystitis Association (2004)

-This book explores the many aspects of IC pain and offers suggestions for relief.

Breaking Through Chronic Pelvic Pain: A Holistic Approach to Relief, by Dr. Jerome Weiss (2019)

-This book describes a holistic approach to treating pelvic pain. It is especially helpful for muscle/myofascial phenotypes.

Facing Pelvic Pain, A Guide for Patients and Their Families, by Elise J.B. De, M.D. and Theodore Stern, M.D. (2020)

-Written by leading experts at Massachusetts General Hospital, it covers many overlapping chronic pain conditions. Has excellent pictures and diagrams as well as a treatment map that allows you to organize all pertinent information in an organized format.

When It Hurts Down There: 15 Proven Techniques to Alleviate Pelvic Pain, by Dr. Angie Stoehr (2018)

-Written by a gynecologist, focuses on pelvic and sexual pain with a comprehensive approach to diagnosing and treating. Covers many causes of pelvic pain in women, besides IC/BPS.

Diet

A taste of the Good Life: A Cookbook for an IC Diet, by Beverley Laumann (1998)

The IC Chef Cookbook, More Than 260 Bladder-Friendly Recipes Shared by Patients Just like You, by Jill H. Osborne, MA (2015)

Confident Choices: Customizing the IC Diet, by Julie Beyer, MA, RD (2010)

-This book outlines how to customize the IC diet to help meet your individual needs. Helps to guide you with an elimination diet.

Confident Choices: A Cookbook for IC and OAB, by Julie Beyer MA, RD (2008)

-Includes over 200 recipes for those with a fussy bladder, whether it is from IC or OAB.

IC-Friendly Summer Eats, by Callie Krajcir, Beverly Levesque, and Kerrie Cole (Sept. 2022)

-Contains over 50 summer recipes. Written by two IC nutritionists and an IC warrior.

Apps to Help You on Your Journey

Bladder Tracker®: This is a free app developed by the IC Network and Natural Approach Nutrition. It tracks symptoms, pain levels, diet, hydration, and sleep quality.

Bladder Pal®: This app lets you track how much you drink, how often you go to the bathroom, and whether you had leakage. The AUA symptom questionnaire is also on the app.

Headspace®: This is an everyday mindfulness and meditation app with great reviews.

Calm®: is an app for both mindfulness and to help with sleep.

Curable®: is an app and healing program that provides patients with evidence-based techniques for chronic pain self-care. This includes cognitive-behavioral therapy, pain reprocessing therapy, guided meditations, visualization, pain science education, and much more. If you would like a six-week free trial, go to my website at www.icjourneytowellness.com.

There are many more apps available that can be helpful as you plan your journey to wellness.

FREE GIFT

Thank you for buying *IC Journey to Wellness*.
I have a free *IC Journey to Wellness* Workbook and Journal that'll
help you on your journey to wellness. Assemble your care team,
keep track of dietary triggers, and more.

Just click below to get it now:
https://icjourneytowellness.com/freebie

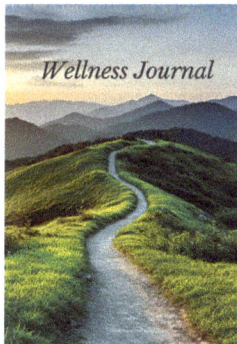

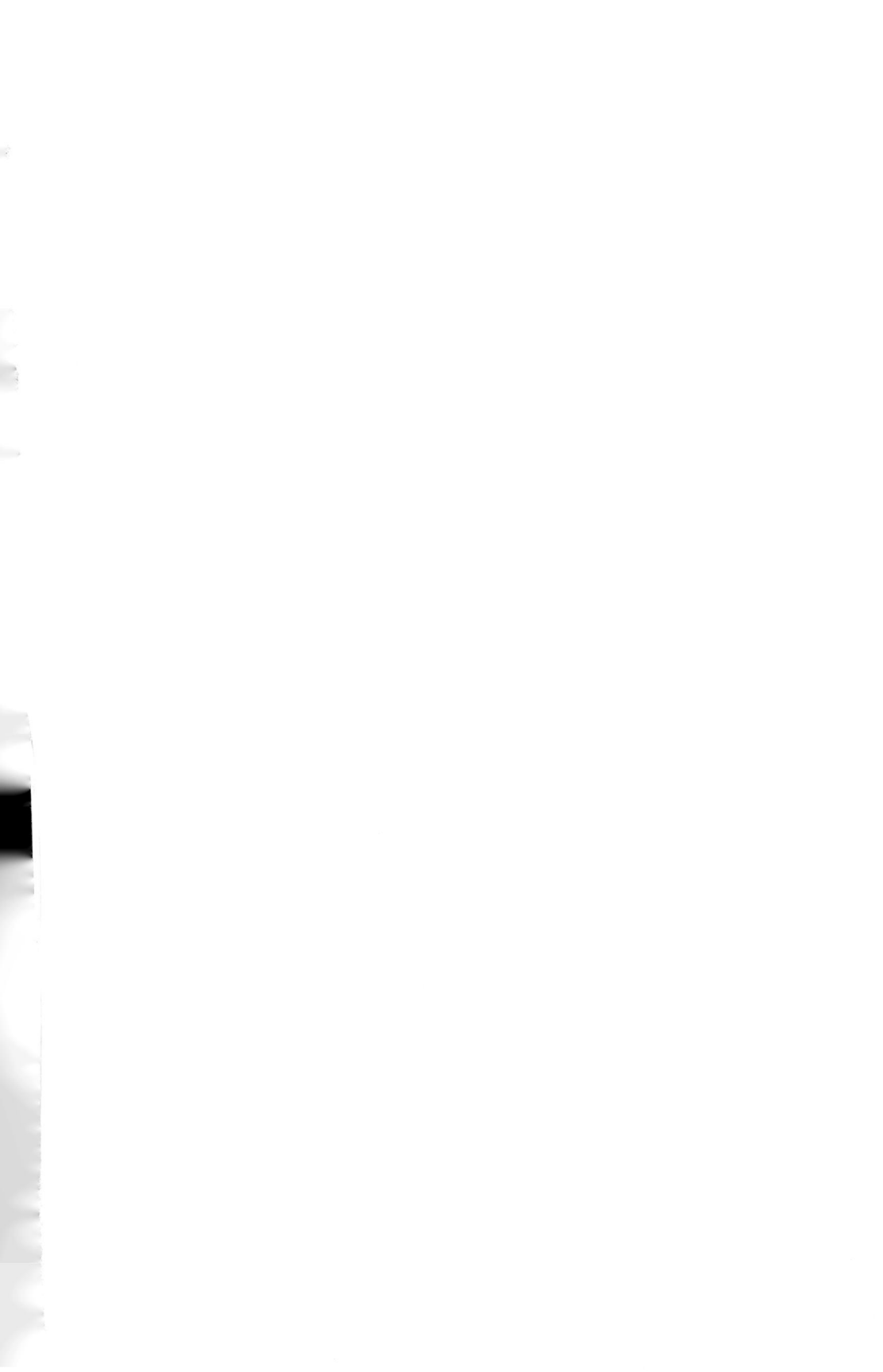

www.ingramcontent.com/pod-product-compliance
Lightning Source LLC
Chambersburg PA
CBHW062128020426
42335CB00013B/1134